ACUPUNCTURE
TREATMENT

SECOND EDITION

ACUPUNCTURE
TREATMENT

SECOND EDITION

SHIN HAK PANG

Translated by James S. BANG, Ph.D.

Lee Business Service
Chicago, IL

Library of Congress Catalog Card Number: 94-93953

ISBN 0-914524-01-1

Printed in the United States of America.

Dong Nam CO. $29.95

2946 N. Lincoln Ave.
Chicago, Illinois 60657

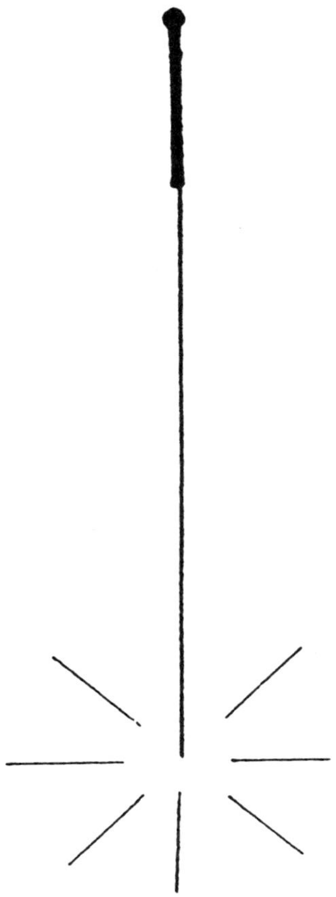

RECOGNITION

Oriental medicine is 5,000 years old;has benefit oriental people throughout those many years.On the other hand modern medicine is much more recent and although continually developing in knowledge has sometimes fell short of its objective at times when oriental medicine has been beneficial.

It is now time for oriental medicine to come into full focus. If it is truly a good and useful medical practice, it will make itself known to the whole world as a harmonious part of the total medical field - A proper balance of ancient oriental medicine involved in a modern medical setting. It will infiltrate as it should because it is needed. Doctors have little faith in Acupuncture because they have scanty knowledge of its concepts.

Rev. Pang have graduated from Tai Han Acupuncture Institute and also studied Acupuncture in Japan and China. Rev. Pang is a professor of the acupuncture science; studying diligently in this oriental art Although has been an ordained minister practicing his theology for many years he has given much to people in need through knowledge and application of Acupuncture during the past 30 years. For the past several years Rev. Pang has researched to tell the proper story of Acupuncture to the western world. His efforts have been trained in the direction of writing a book that could present history and techniques to anyone who wished to comprehend the science and philosophy of Acupuncture.

It is quite astonishing that this fine written work has developed without anyone's knowledge of its progress to completion, the final works in completion being truly
comprehensive and potentially useful in our world.

This book "Acupuncture (Treatment)", I believe is so much of a contribution to the western world's library of medicine that I, a man who has spent a large part of my life studying Acupuncture, its philosophy and application; heartily endorse its presentation to the world. I feel compelled to add my congratulation s to Rev. Pang for it's writing.

The book is complete in its information. The patient who uses this "Acupuncture(Treatment)" book will be benefited.

Technical people wishing to comprehend and learn Acupuncture should make this book an initial must in their studies.

Congratulations for this fine book Rev. Pang and thank you.

Chang Bin Lee
President, World Congress of Acupuncture
President, Korea Academic Society of Acupuncture
Dean & Prof. Oriental Medical college of Won Kuang University, Seoul, Korea
Professor, Loyola University Stritch School of Medicine, Chicago, Illinois U.S.A.

May,1973

PREFACE

The recent journalistic reports about astonish-ing performances of an Oriental art of medical treatment, the so-called Acupuncture, seem to have caused much amusement as well as considerable suspicion among many American people. How is it possible that patients can undergo surgical operations exclusively by Acupuncture anesthesia involving such vital organs as heart, lung, or brain, in full consciousness, while the patients drink fruit juices or exchange conversation with the operating surgeons? How can the deaf be cured by the Acupuncture treatment alone - recovering normal hearing ability and speech? How can an acute appendicitis be cured without any conventional medical operation? Can we really believe that many other ailments, normally considered very difficult or impossible to cure by the current medical practices, can be cured by Acupuncture alone?

The reports of the eyewitnesses, however, are so authentic and realistic that we can not simply dismiss the incontrovertible results of the Acupuncture treatments as merely superstition, mystery, or even fraud. The medical significance of Acupuncture is so extensive that we can not simply ignore or overlook its important role. Accordingly, we have to know something about it, if Acupuncture is to be applied legitimately as a sound medical practice.

This manuscript is, therefore, designed to provide the basic understanding, insight, and knowledge about Acupuncture. The difficulty, however, rests in the fact that Acupuncture is based on a principle of Oriental philosophy, which is almost totally alien to the Western scientific community. Much efforts have been expended in various parts of the world to develop scientific explanation and to provide proof for Acupuncture, but none of these efforts appear to be satisfactory up to date. The author has the conviction that a sound scientific Western society can be formulated only if it is based on the Ion theory as explained and elaborated in the following chapters.

This book, which was originally planned five years ago before leaving Korea, is mainly based on the lectures on Acupuncture delivered at the International Christian Seminary in Seoul, Korea, for the purpose of training students of Acupuncture, who would work in the field of Christian ministry. The recent arrival of Mr.B.K.Lee, the foremost authority on Acupuncture, from Korea and the author's two sons, Un Song,M.D. and Hyo Song,M.D. made it possible for him to resume the work in completing this manuscript. The illustration were kindly provided by Mr.Dorian Figura. The author is very grateful to Professor James S. Bang, Department of Sociology, Anthropology, and Psychology at the University of Wisconsin - Sheboygan, who read, corrected and translated many parts of this manuscript.

Through my twenty-seven years of experience as teacher of Oriental Medicine, I have found many difficulties and inconveniences on teaching Acupuncture's meridian points to my American students. Students with limited or no understanding of Chinese, Japanese or Korean language have been required to memorize the hundreds of meridian points not by meaning, but rather through letter-number code. Since there have been no comprehensive Acupuncture texts which address this inconsistency,I have decided to publish a revised edition of Acupuncture Treatment which provides English translations of meridian points.

This revised edition is in response to my

students' frustrations and my hope for an international understanding of Acupuncture points. I have translated the original points name used by the Oriental people to the nearest English translation. I hope that through this revised edition, many American students would find this text thorough and helpful in their studies.

S.H.P.

INTRODUCTION

In the medical treatment, "Acupuncture" is the first, "Moxabusion", the second, "Medicine", the third.

-an ancient Chinese saying-

1. The Discovery of Acupuncture by the American people. When President Nixon and other American representatives visited China last March, they found in certain Chinese hospitals one of the most unusual phenomena. Witnessing the most delicate and dangerous operations such as surgeries of heart, lung, and brain, the distinguished visitors were fascinated by the fact that patients on the operating table were clearly awake in full consciousness of the operation. The patients were drinking fruit-juice and exchanging words with the operating doctors during the entire period of operation. Yet it was quite clear, and without any doubt at all, that the patients were experiencing no pain whatsoever. It was no wonder that the visitors were very much impressed by such unusual events, since they had almost no comprehensive idea about the effectiveness of Acupuncture. In other words, those patients were anesthetized by the delicate use of acupuncture. By inserting needles gently into the skin at certain parts of ears, hands, legs, or neck in human body, the patients were anesthetized without any medication or chemicals. Furthermore, the visitors had witnessed and learned that polio, rheumatism, schizophrenia, acute appendicitis, deafs, mutes, and etc. In fact, Acupuncture treatment can be applied to almost all the diseases and illnesses known to man.

2. Among the American visitors was Mr.Reston, a well-known editorial columnist and vice president of the New York Times., whose reports were recently televised to the American people. Subsequently, it

well-known editorial columnist and vice president of the New York Times., whose reports were recently televised to the American people. Subsequently, it was reported that more than six hundred persons suffering from various ailments made trips from European countries to the mainland China for medical treatments by Acupuncture. In England, France, Germany, and Russia as well as in Asian countries, intensive interest has been generated towards the study and development of Acupuncture treatment. In the United States, President Nixon has commissioned a group of respectable American physicians to go to the mainland China for observation and evaluation of Acupuncture treatment, since it was felt that the American Public should be informed of the significance of this ancient practice - 5,000 years old art, which needs its Western exposure. In the mainland China, Acupuncture anesthetic has been extensively employed instead of chemical anesthetics which might cause some deleterious effects on the human body. The author believes that no part of the world should be shy away from seeking the truth, especially in regard to Acupuncture.

3. It has been twenty-five years since the author began the offering of Acupuncture treatment to many different patients;twenty years in Korea and, subsequently, five years in the Chicago area. He has been practicing it as a Christian minister - not as a professional physician. Acupuncture treatment can be performed so simply that one does not need any medicines, or elaborate facilities. The patients are usually persons whose ailments are thought incurable. The author has seen so many patients experiencing happiness and bliss at having their ailments cured by this ancient art of Acupuncture. In this monograph, the author intends to explain systematically how Acupuncture treatments are given efficiently and effectively. The treatments are so simple, and without any danger, that any person, not only physicians but

also the patients themselves, can apply the treatment only if its users are competently trained in the use of Acupuncture. The author believes strongly that it is one crucial part of his ministerial role to pursue the "gospel" of Acupuncture while residing in the United States.

WHAT IS ACUPUNCTURE?

Acupuncture, in brief, is an ancient art of healing through the use of special needles. For Acupuncture treatment, the only required tools are needles and the knowledge of their application and effects. No chemical medicines nor any other means are require. There are nine different kinds of needles being employed currently. When these needles are penetrated into the skin at various depths, very little pain is felt - far less pain or irritation than the one felt with conventional injections. In fact, Acupuncture needles are usually less painful than injection needles, which are usually sharper. The needles are sterilized just like the conventional injection needles.

On the surface of the human body there are about 650 points where Acupuncture needles can be safely inserted. The selection of particular points for Acupuncture treatment is very crucial in determining the success or failure of a treatment. The prerequisite to the accurate selection of points is the correct diagnosis of the ailment; where it is manifested, and how it originated as well as what is the nature of the ailment. These and other relevant questions are raised and responded in terms of the classical oriental philosophy and practice, which are very complex and, accordingly, require much practical experiences.

Diagnosis is usually made by feeling the pulse with two fingers, and then, through inspection of patient's countenance, voice, and through questioning of the patient. Before inserting needles one must locate the most sensitive points, which can be identified by pressing with his fingers, and, then, the needles are to be inserted at those points. The first insertion of these needles would bring some positive effects immediately on the patient. He would feel better, relieved, and consequently, believe that some more treatment like this will alleviate his ailment.

TABLE OF CONTENTS

YIN, YANG AND ACUPUNCTURE

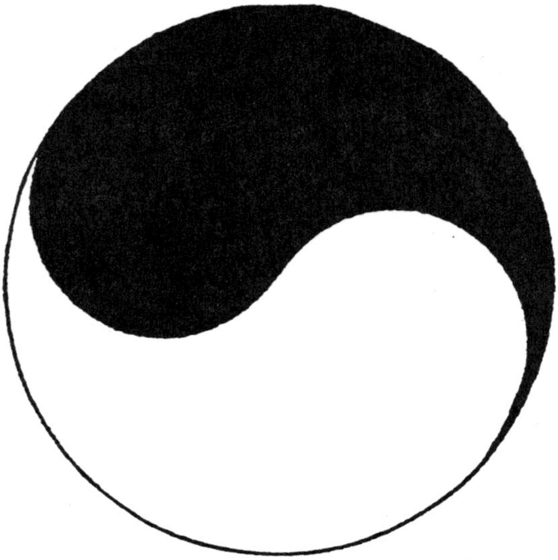

YIN MEANS THE DARK, COLD, WEAK, FEMALE, NEGATIVE FORCE.

YANG MEANS THE LIGHT, HOT, STRONG, MALE, POSITIVE FORCE.

BREATHED?

"AND THE LORD GOD FORMED MAN OF THE DUST OF THE GROUND* AND BREATHED INTO HIS NOSTRILLS THE BREATH OF LIFE: AND MAN BECAME A LIVING SOUL."

- Genesis 2 : 7

Fourteen Symbols of Meridian

1.	Lungs	L - (= =)	Greater Yin
2.	Large Intestine	LI - (≡)	Sun-Light Yang
3.	Stomach	S - (≡)	Sun-Light Yang
4.	Spleen	SP - (= =)	Greater Yin
5.	Heart	H - (= =)	Lesser Yin
6.	Small Intestine	SI - (=)	Greater Yang
7.	Bladder	B - (=)	Greater Yang
8.	Kidney	K - (= =)	Lesser Yin
9.	Circulation-Sex	CS - (≡ ≡)	Absolute Yin
10.	Triple Warmer	T - (= =)	Lesser Yang
11.	Gall Bladder	GB - (= =)	Lesser Yang
12.	Liver	LV - (≡ ≡)	Absolute Yin
13.	Governing Vessel	GV - (=)	Greater Yang
14.	Conception Vessel	CV - (= =)	Greater Yin

1. LUNGS 手太陰肺經 L - (==) Greater Yin

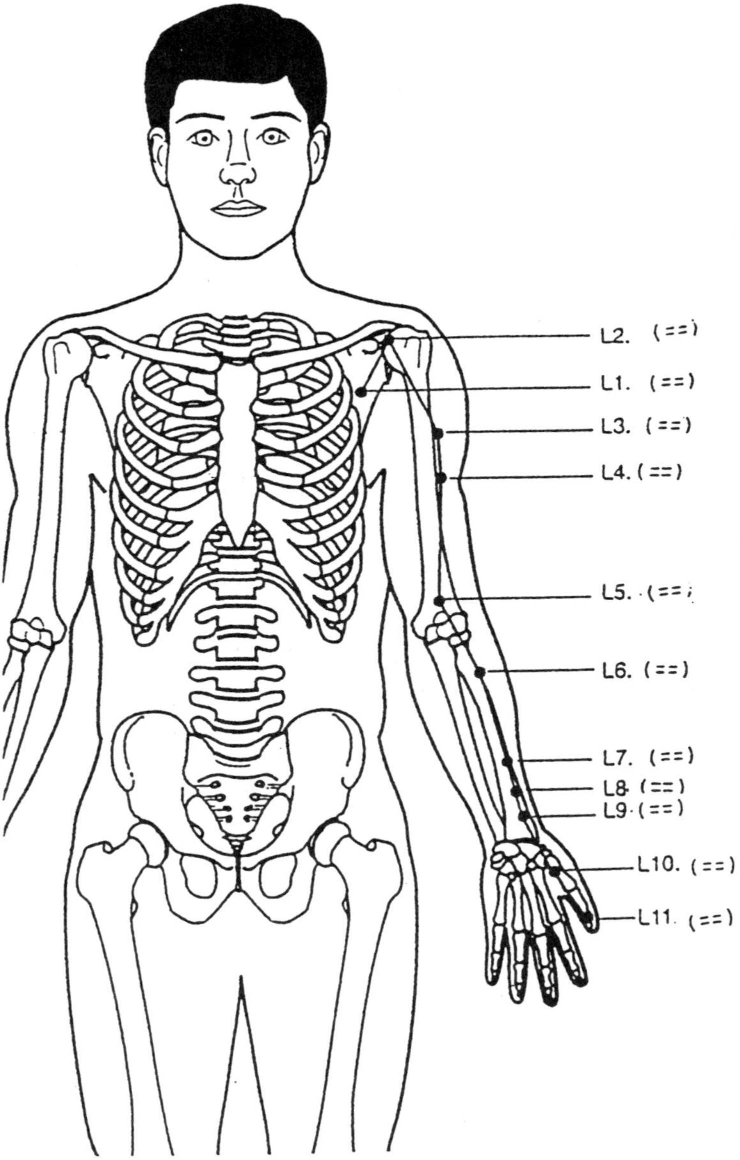

2. LARGE INTESTINE 手陽明大腸經 LI - (☰) Sun-Light Yang

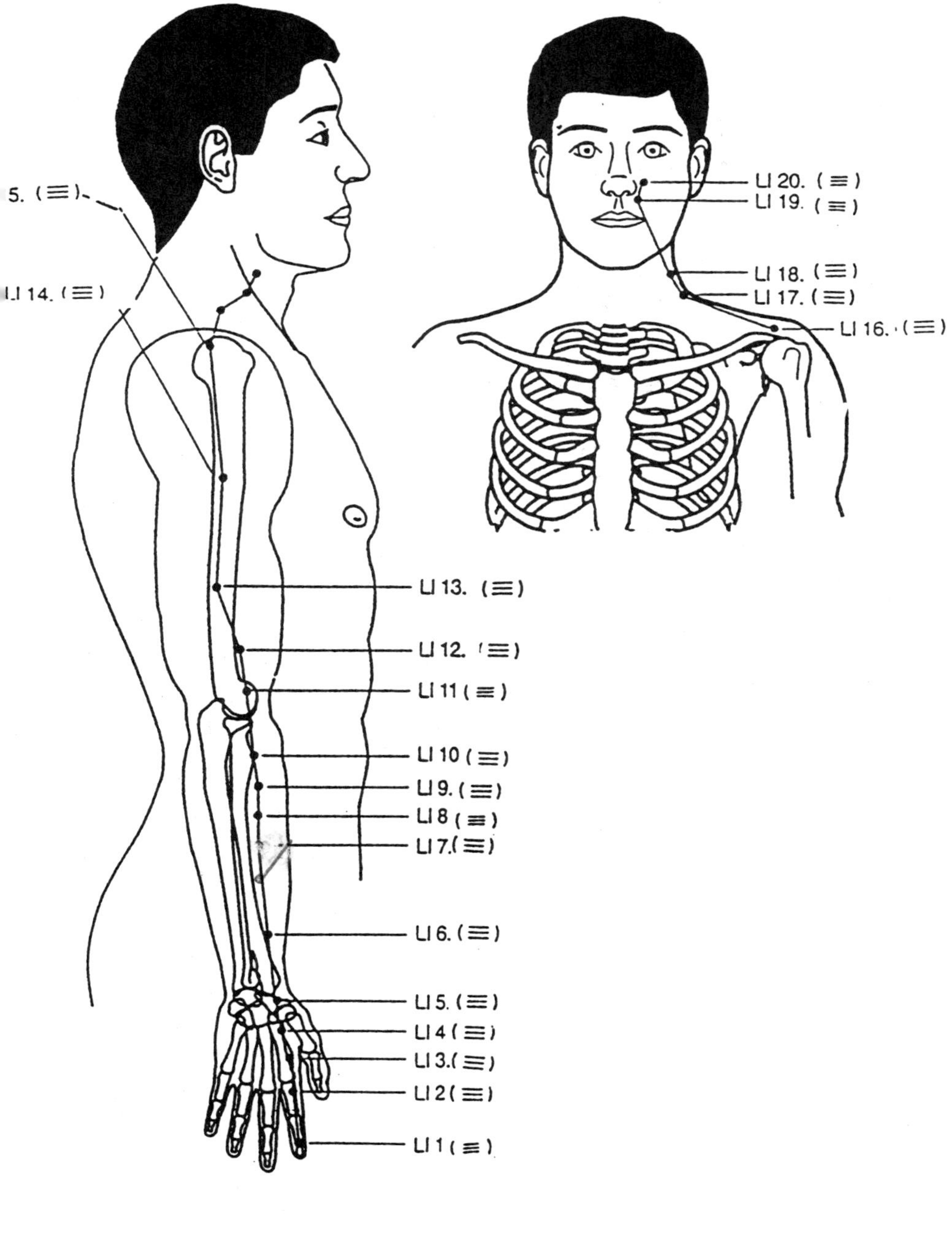

3. STOMACK 足陽明胃經 S - (☰) Sun-Light Yang

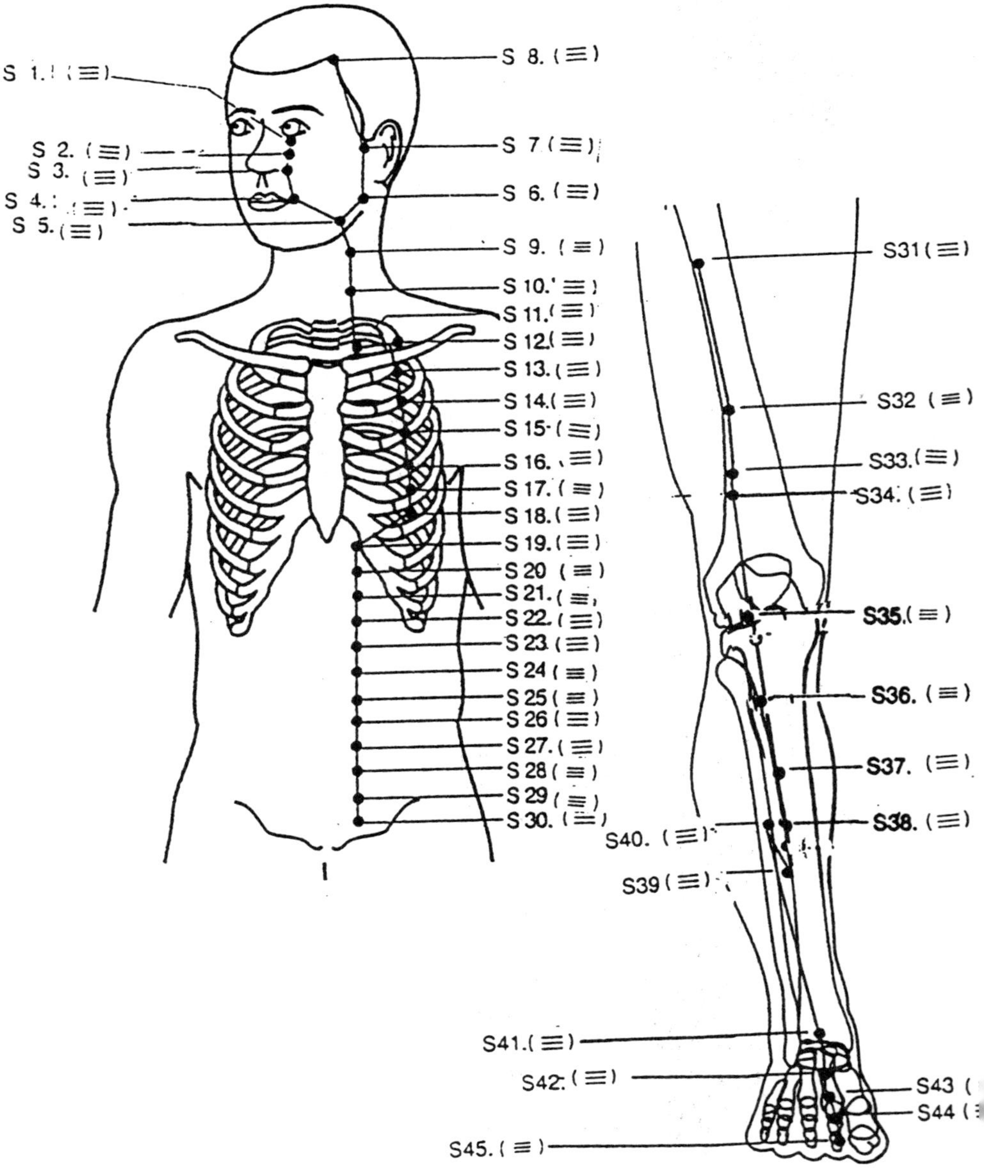

4. SPLEEN 足太陰脾經 SP - (==) Greater Yin

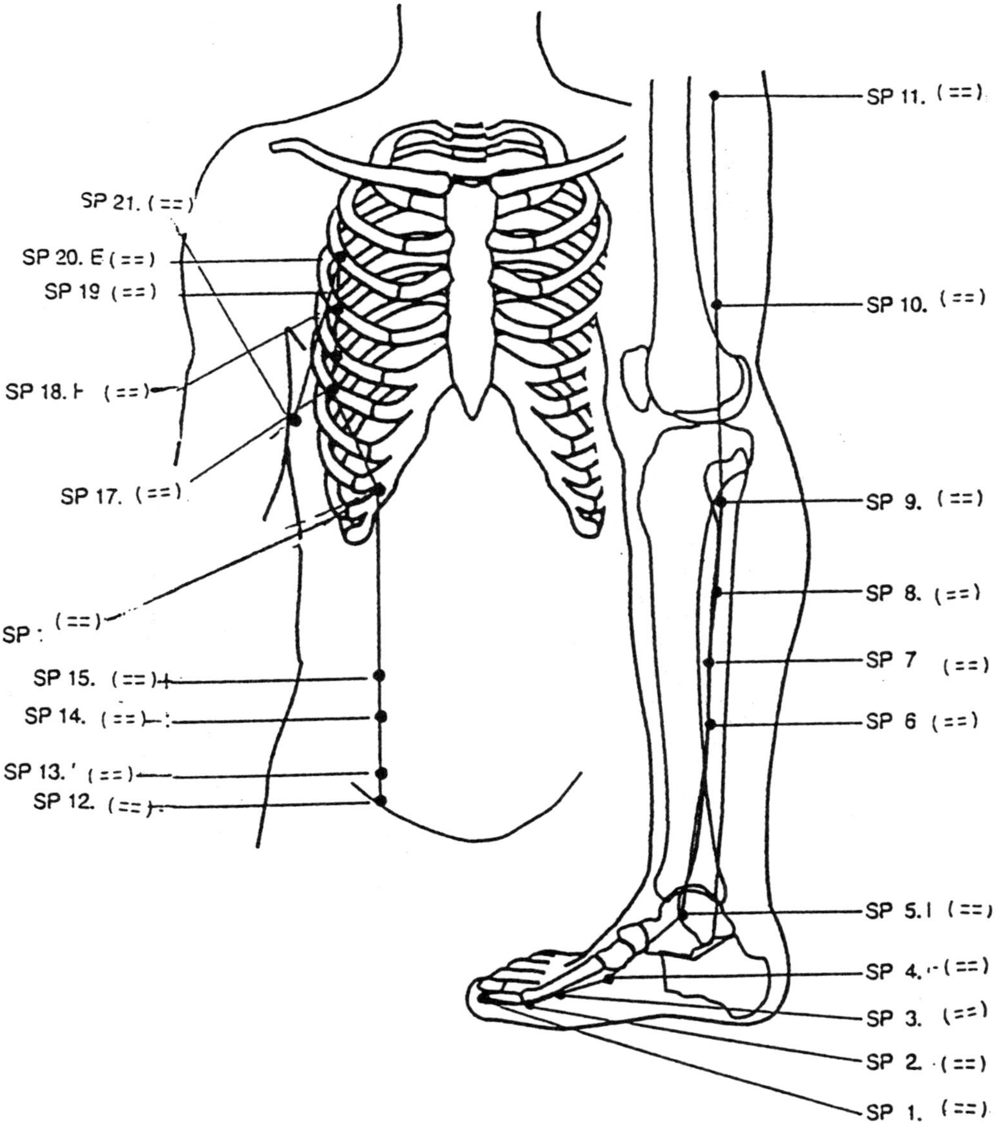

5. HEART 手少陰心經 H - (==) Lesser Yin

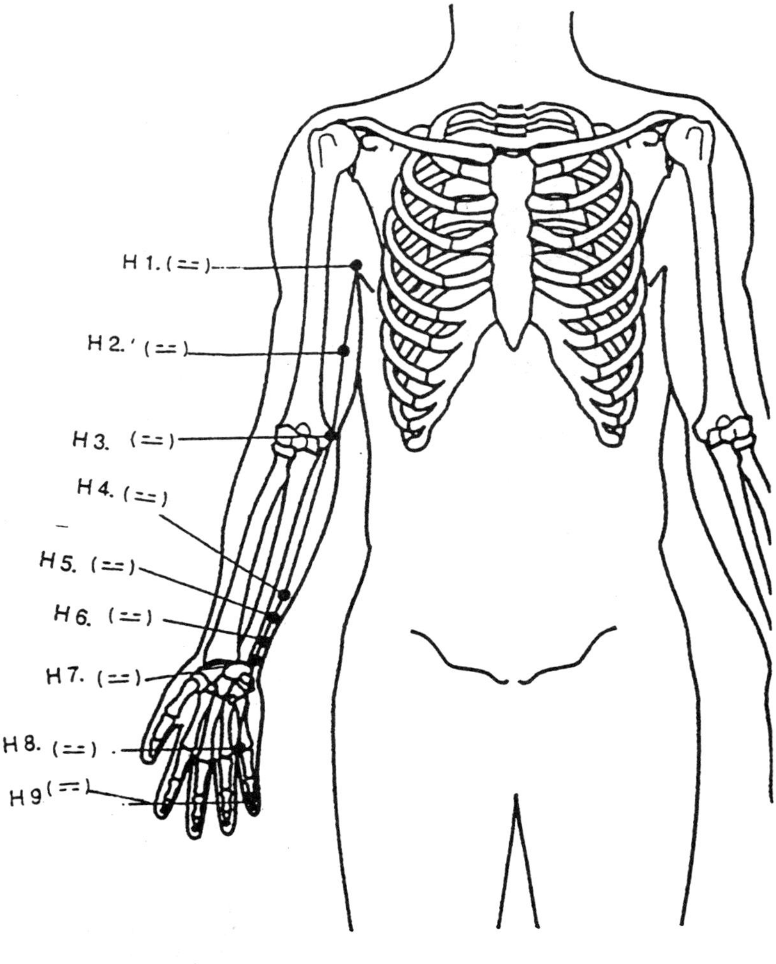

6. SMALL INTESTINE 手太陽小腸經 SI - (二) GREATER Yang

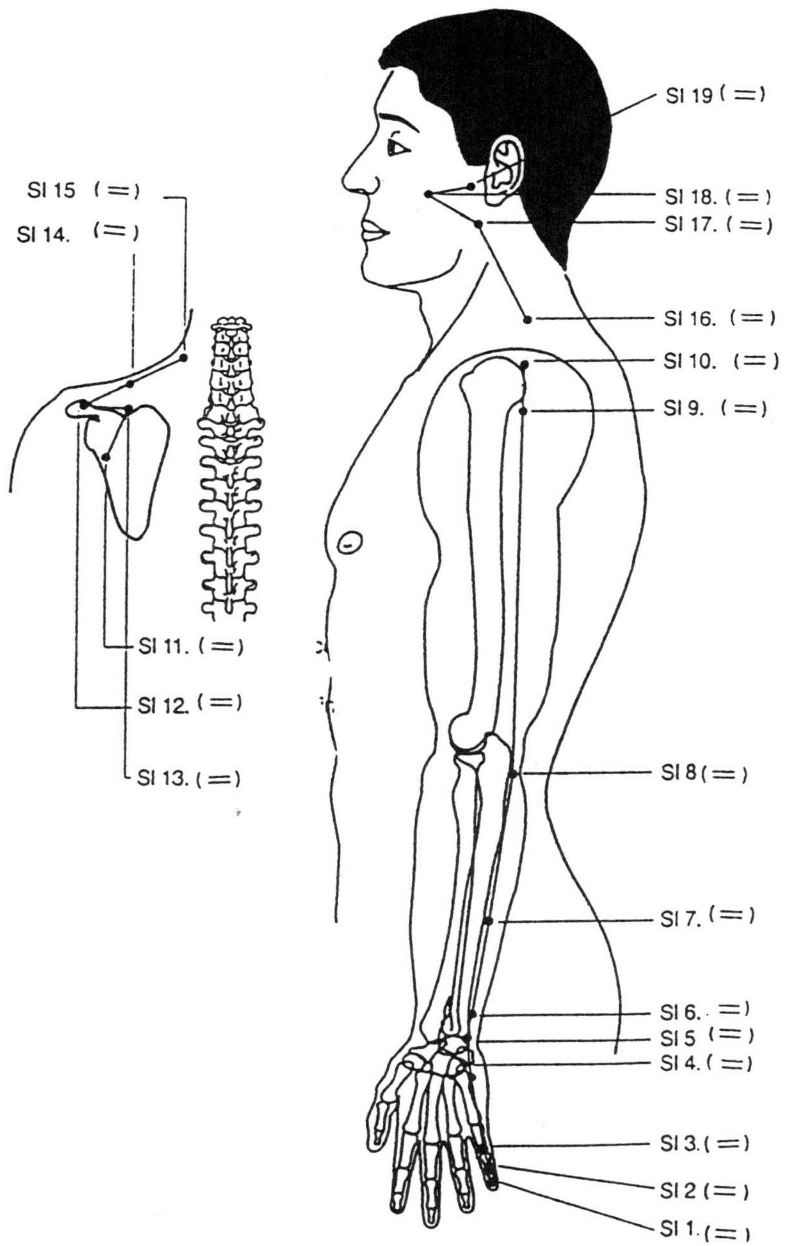

7. BLADDER 足太陽膀胱經 B - (=) Greater Yang

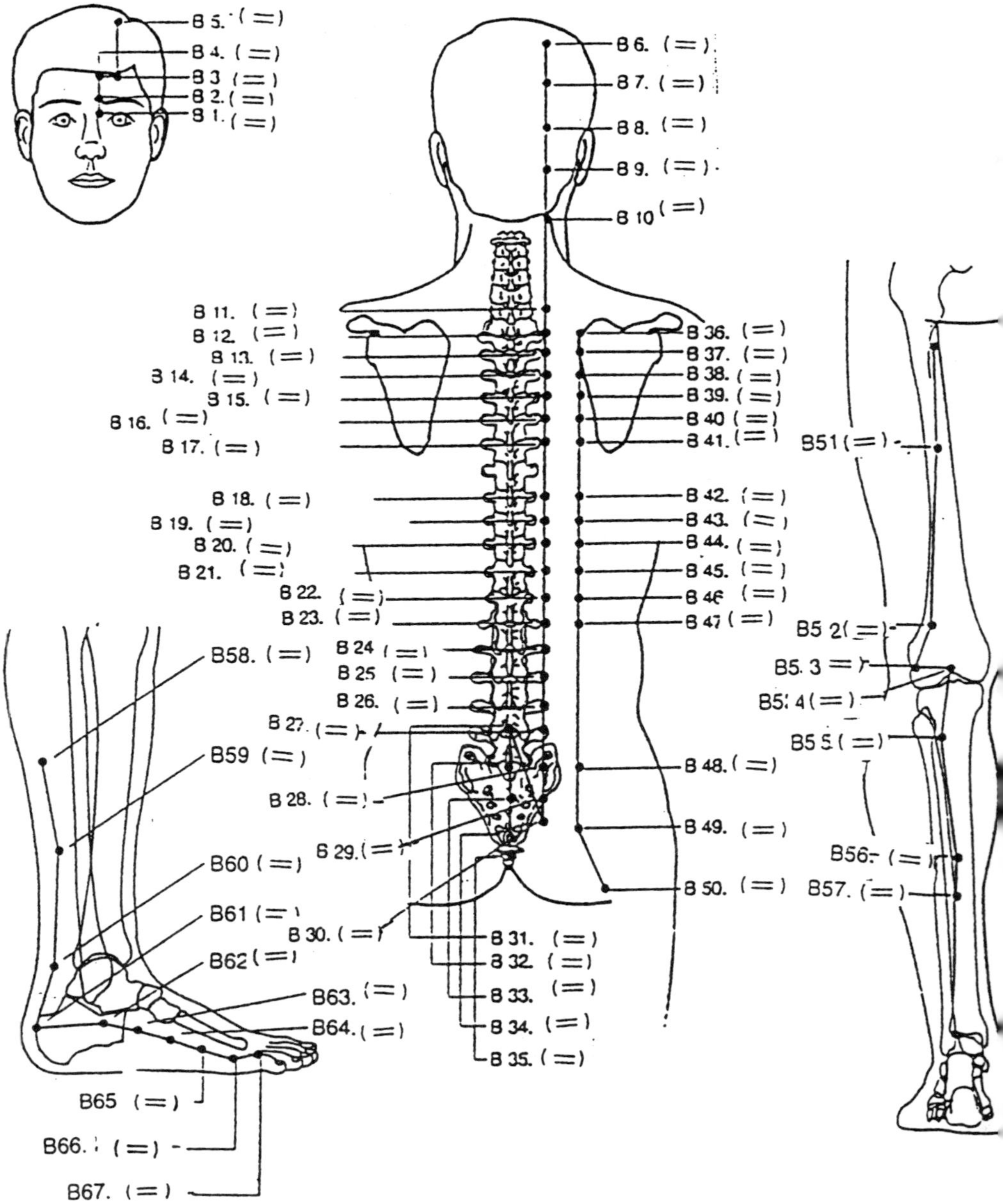

KIDNEY 足少陰腎經 K - (==) Lesser Yin

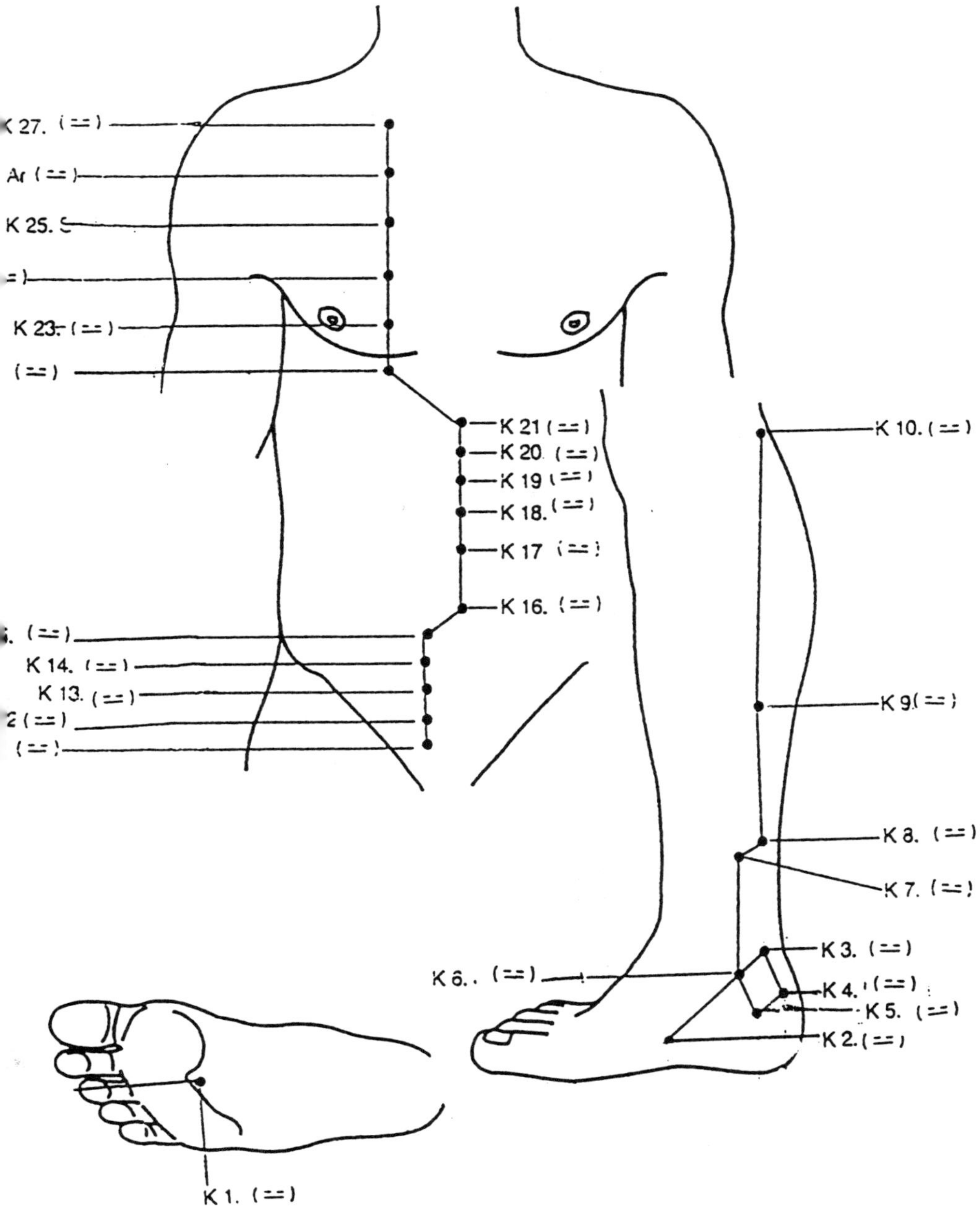

9. CIRCULATION-SEX 手厥陰心包經 P - (☰☰) Absolute Yin

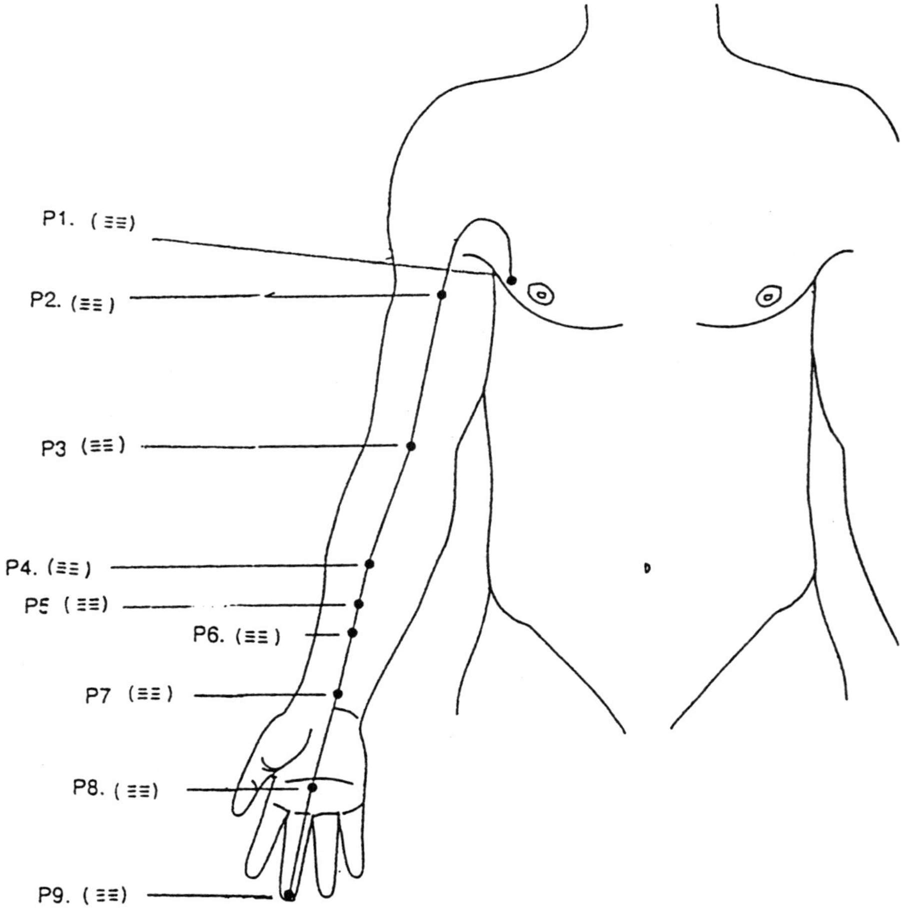

10. TRIPLE WARMER 手少陽三焦經 T - (☳) Lesser Yang

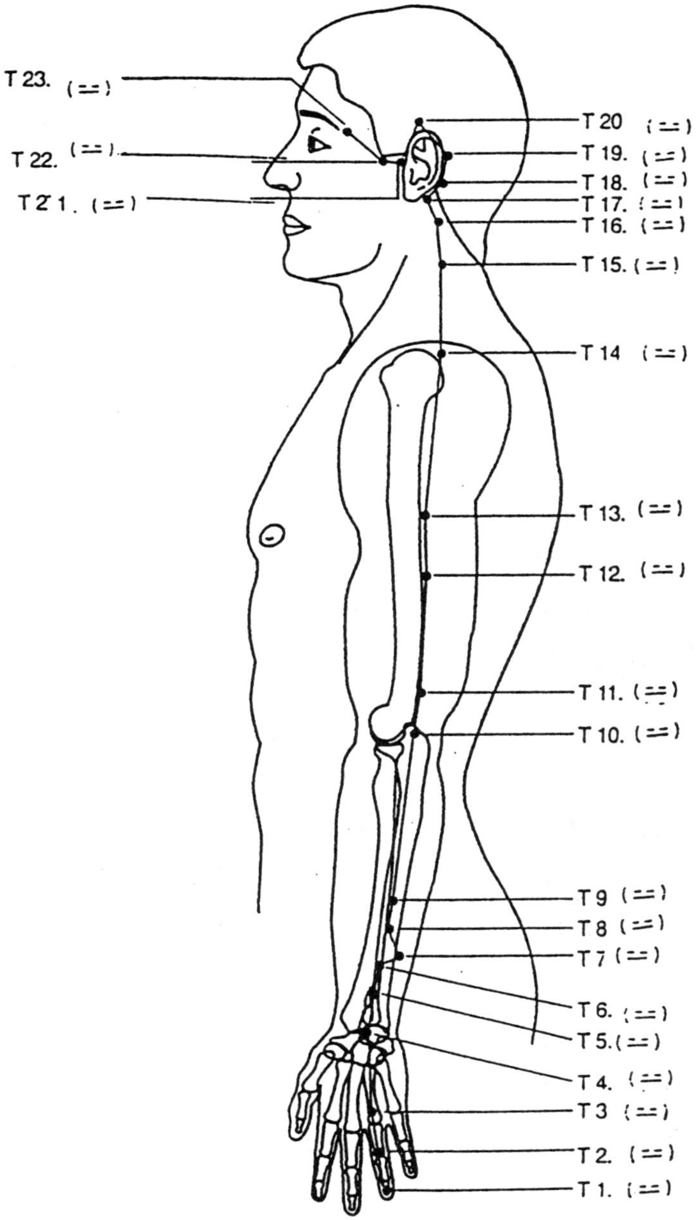

11. GALL BLADDER 足少陽胆經 GB - (==) Lesser Yang

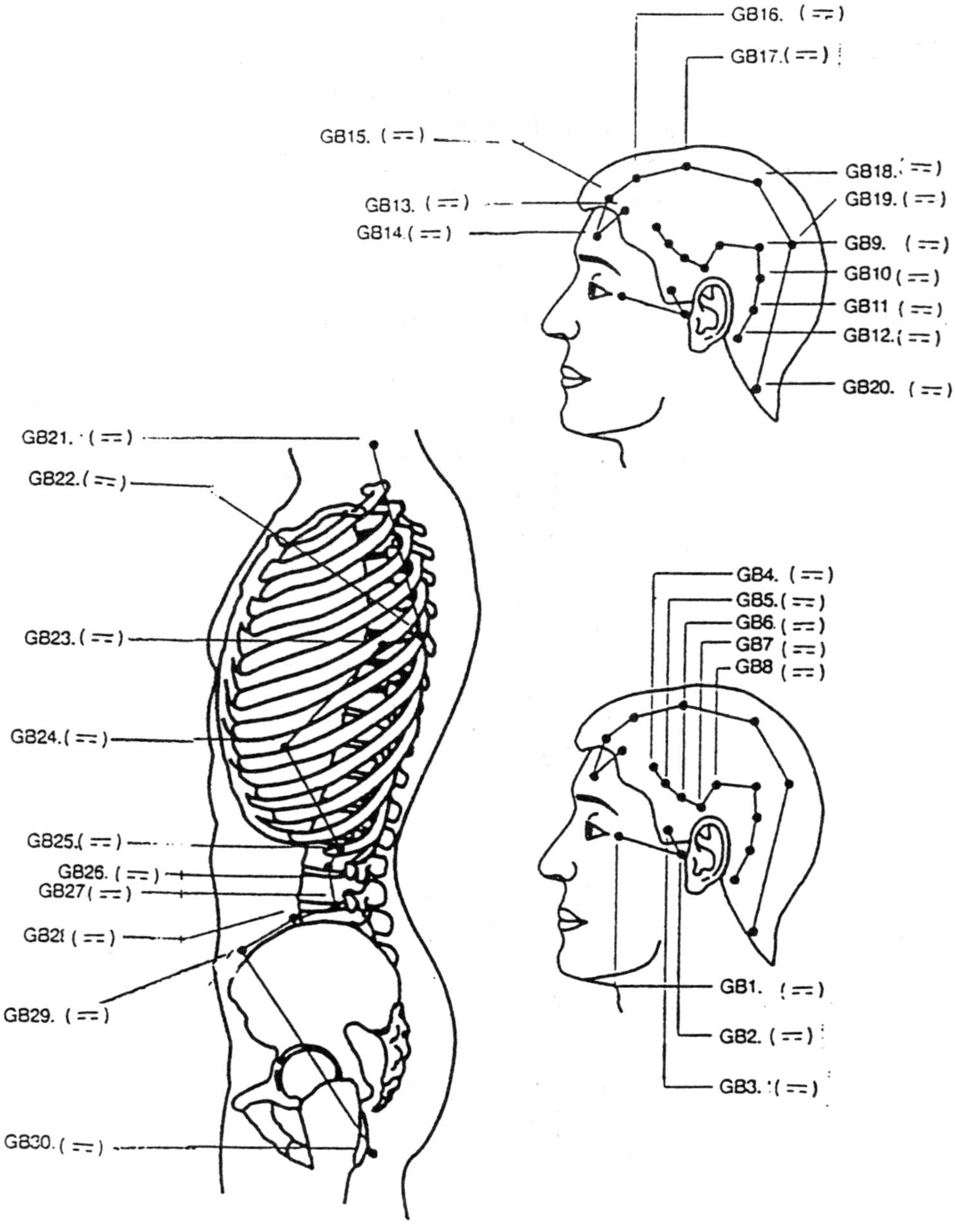

12. LIVER 足厥陰肝經 LV - (☳) Absolute Yin

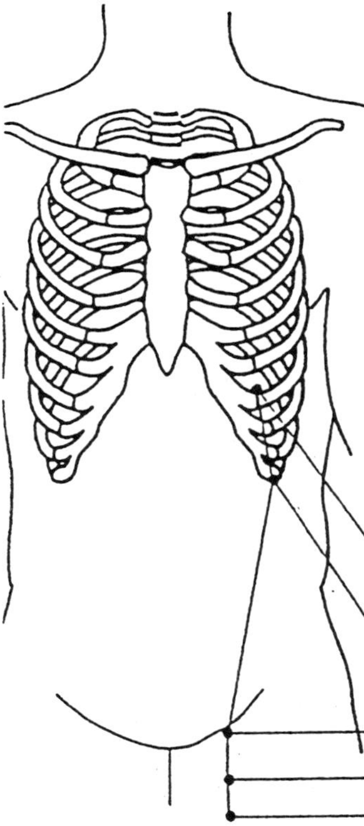

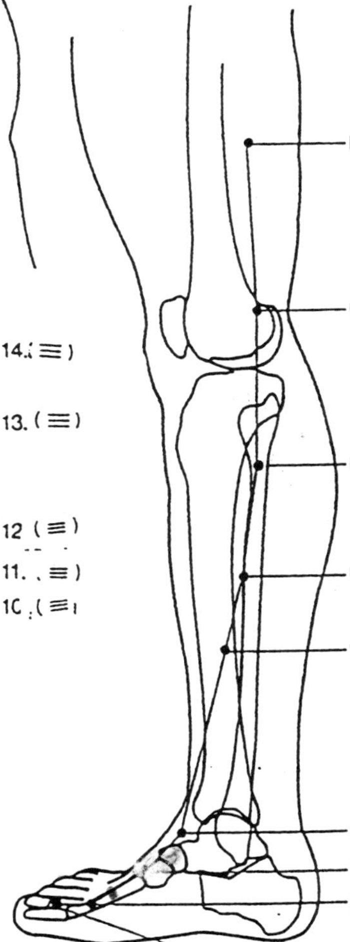

13. GOVERNING VESSEL 督 脈 GV - (═) Greater Yang

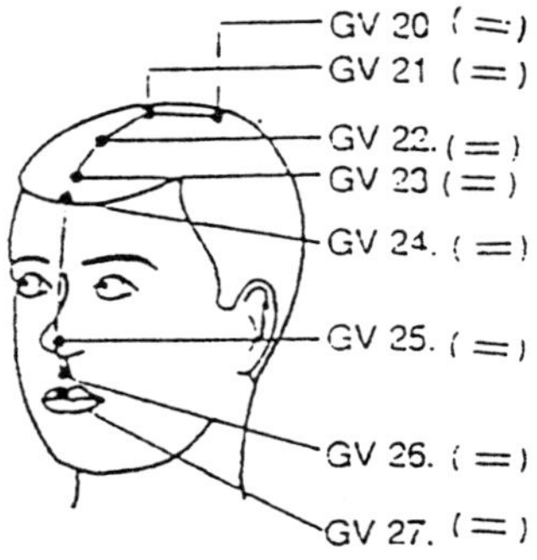

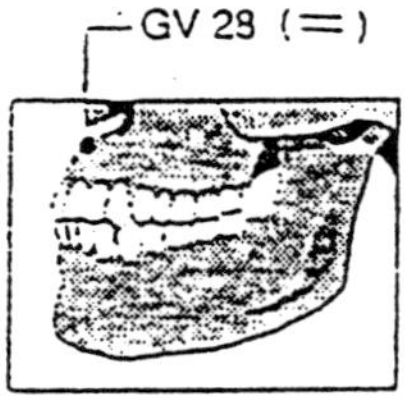

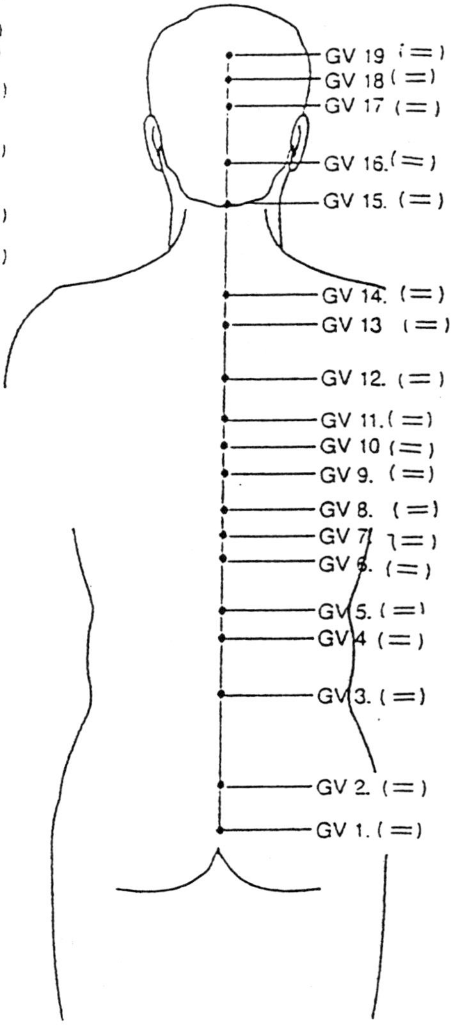

14. CONCEPTION VESSEL 督 脈 CV - (==) Greater Yin

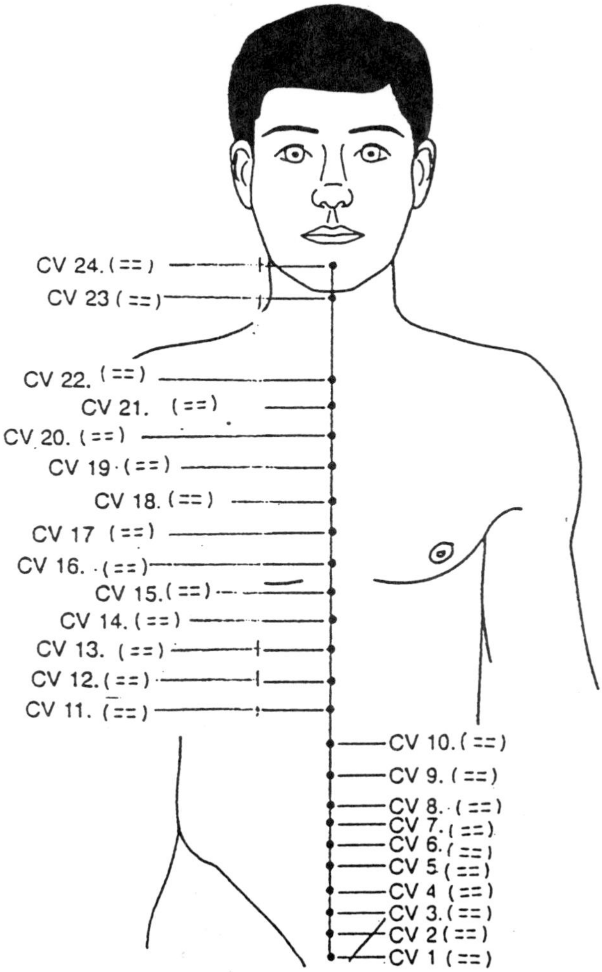

"HOW TO MEASURE ACUPUNCTURE"

THE INCHES WE USE IN THIS BOOK ARE THE MEASURES THEY USE IN THE ORIENT FOR ACUPUNCTURE. ALSO THEY ARE CALLED "CHI". "CHI" IS VERY MUCH LIKE INCH. "CHI" IS ALMOST THE SAME AS INCH IN LENGTH.

1. When you look at Figure # 1, you see the middle finger. The finger is in banded position. The space of the banded finger is about one inch long.

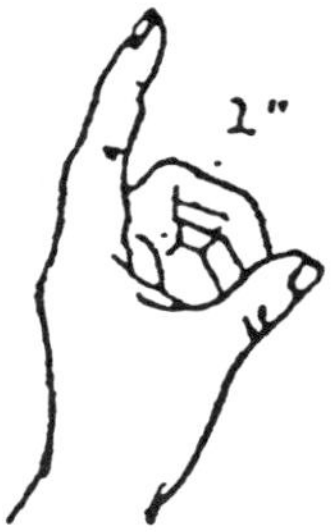

Figure # 1

2. When you look at Figure # 2, you see the thumb, The thickest part of the thumb is one inch wide.

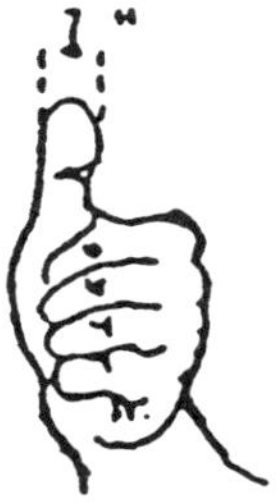

Figure # 2

3. When you look at Figure # 3, you see a picture showing the distance between two ears. When you measure the distance between two ears (using back side) and, then, divide it by nine(9), your answer is about one inch.

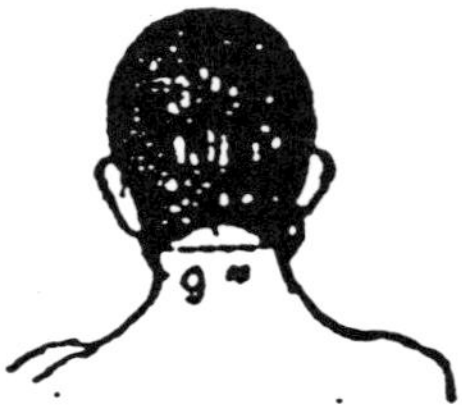

Figure # 3

4. When you look at Figure #4, you see a man's head showing side ways. From B = 2 to GV = 23 the distance is three (3) inches long. And from GV = 23 to GV = 16 it is twelve (12) inches long. Also from top of the back neck (between where hairs are and the neck) to GV = 13 the distance is three(3) inches.

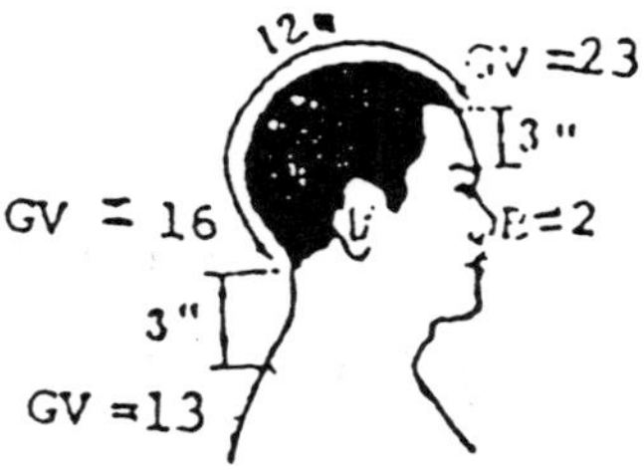

Figure # 4

5. Figure #5 shows two fingers, whose width is 1.5 inches.

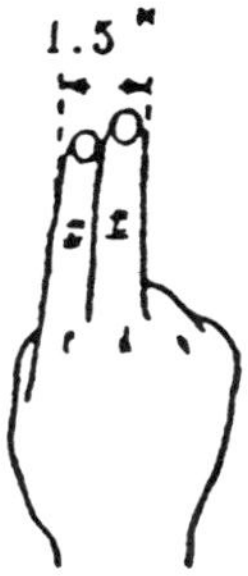

Figure # 5

6. In Figure #6 you see your fingers together. They are about three (3) inches wide.

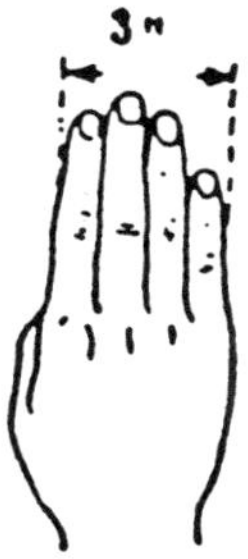

Figure # 6

POSTURES FOR ACUPUNCTURE TREATMENT

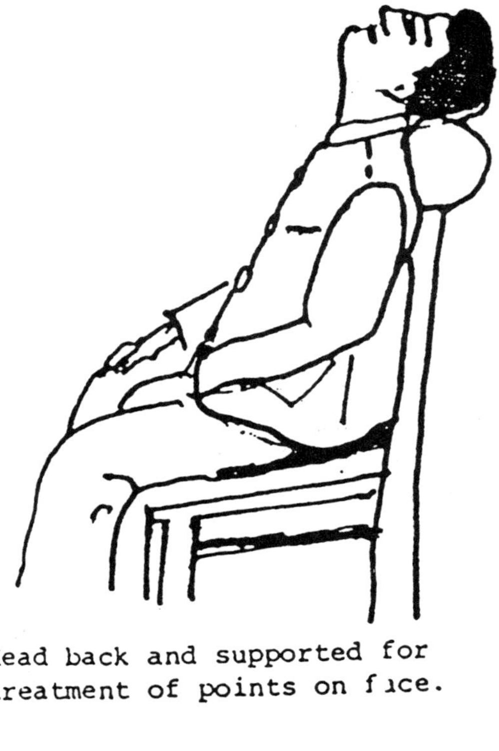

Head back and supported for treatment of points on f ice.

POSTURES FOR ACUPUNCTURE TREATMENT

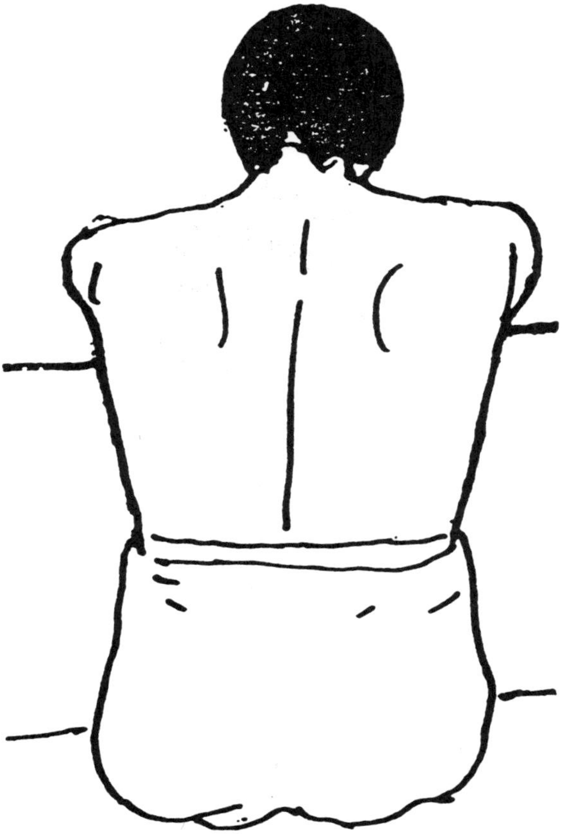

Sitting Position: Resting on arms for treatment of back or neck.

POSTURES FOR ACUPUNCTURE TREATMENT

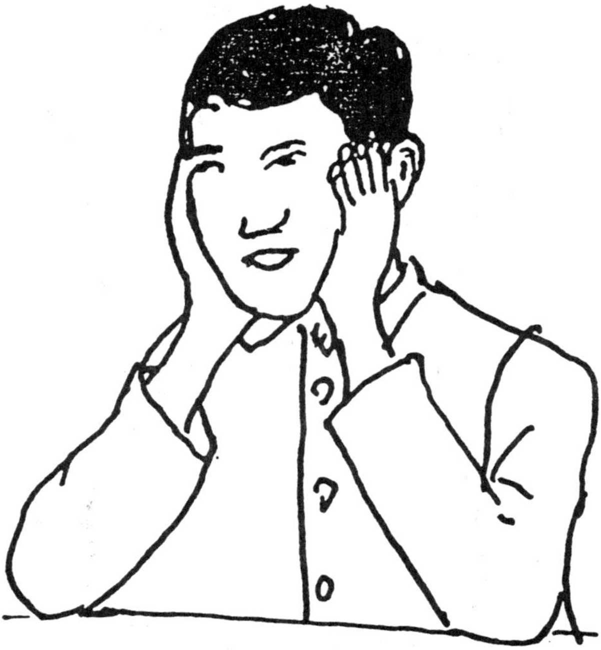

Head supported on hands

(for treatment of points on the forehead)

POSTURES FOR ACUPUNCTURE TREATMENT

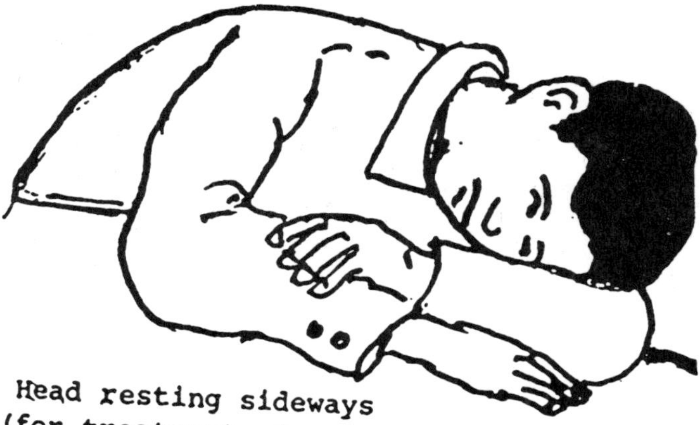

Head resting sideways
(for treatment of points on ear or neck).

POSTURES FOR ACUPUNCTURE TREATMENT

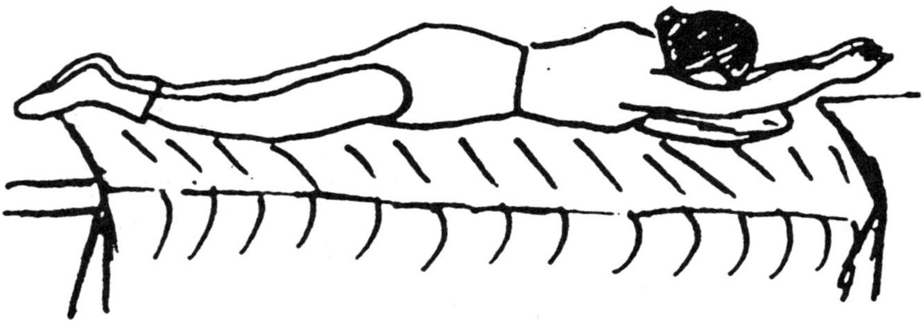

Lying on Stomach: For treatment on the back and hip.

POSTURES FOR ACUPUNCTURE TREATMENT

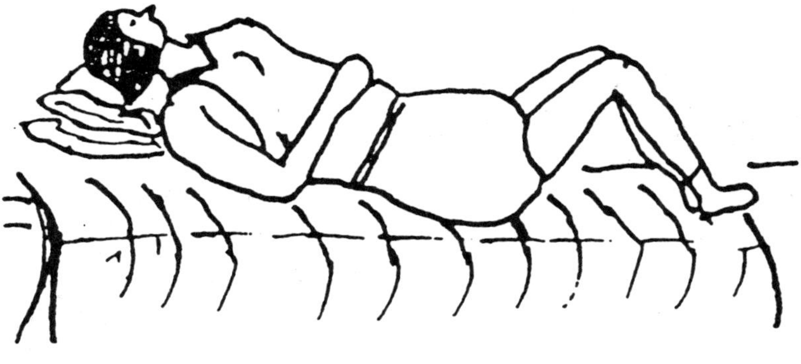

Lying-on-back Position: For treatment on the stomach and legs.

POSTURES FOR ACUPUNCTURE TREATMENT

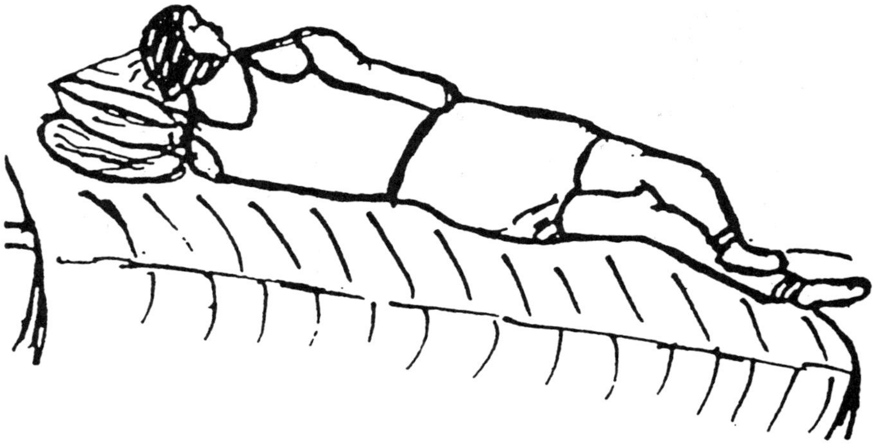

LYING SIDE WAY POSITION

(FOR TREATMENT ON THE HIP AND LEGS)

-DISINFECTION-

. Prier to their application, the needles and case must be sterilized in boiling water for 30 minutes and disinfected with 2-3% of Cresol liquid or 50-70% of alcohol.

. Acupuncurist must disinfect his hands throughly with 2-3% of Cresol liquid or 50-70% of alcohol before treatments.

. The points on the patient's body, where Acupuncture needles are to be applied, must be cleaned with 2-3% of Cresol liquid or 50-70% of alcohol. You must use the medically approved absorbent cotton when you disinfect or clean the Acupuncture points.

isposable Acupuncture needles are mass produced n the United States, so that it is highly ecommended that the used Acupuncture needle hould preferrably be disposed of in order to afeguard the patients.

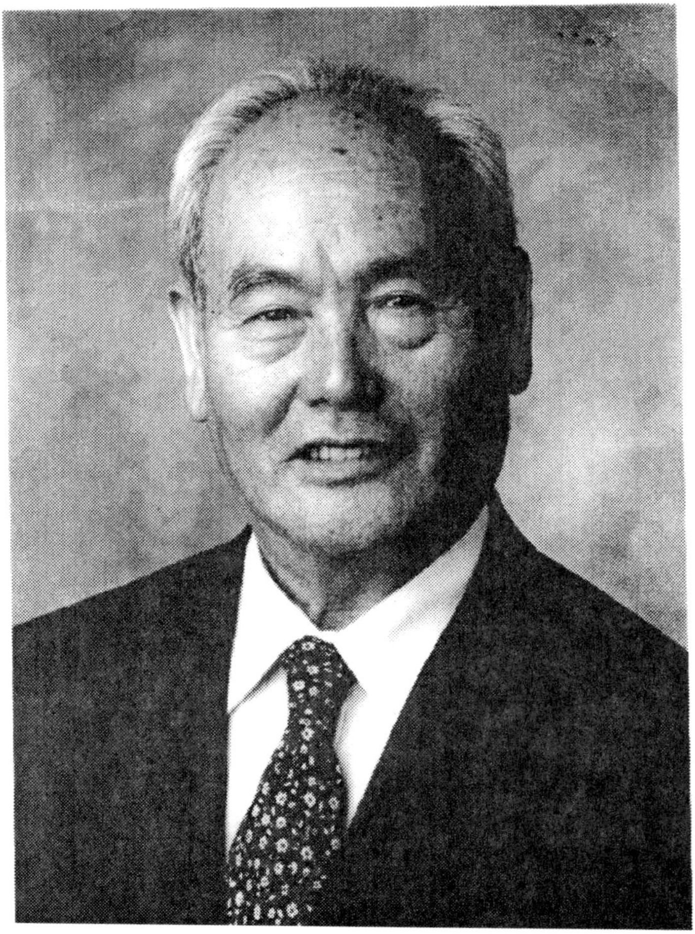

THE AUTHOR COMPARING THE CHART SHOWING MERIDIANS AND HUMAN MODEL SHOWING ACUPUNCTURE POINTS AND COURSES OF MERIDIANS.

CHAPTER I

GENERAL AILMENTS

CHAPTER I
GENERAL AILMENTS

1. HEMIPLEGIA(PART 1)

Hemiplegia is the paralysis of one side of the human body caused by the after-effect of cerebral hemorrhage.

a. Acupunctural Points To Be Used:

Shoulder Well,Wind Pond,Shoulder Bone,Arm Three Miles,Outer Gate,Jumping Circle, Wind Market,Leg Three Miles,Dissolve Stream are used for the needle-insertion:

(1)Shoulder Well(GB.21, Figure FA 1):
Located at the midpoint of the shoulder.

(2)Wind Pond(GB.20, Figure FA 1);
See the Section on Neurasthenia.

(3)Shoulder Bone(LI.15, Figure FA 1):
Located at the arm-shoulder joint on each side.

(4)Arm Three Miles(LI.10, Figure FA 1):
Located two inches down from the elbow on the exterior side.

(5)Outer Gate(T.5, Figure FA 1):
Located between the two bones two inches up from the wrist on the exterior side of the arm.

(6)Jumping Circle(GB.30, Figure FA 1):
Located at each side of the hip.

(7)Leg Samri(S.36, Figure FA 1):
Located under the knee.
See the Section on Neurasthenia.

(8) Dissolve Stream(S.41, Figure FA 1):
Located on the front ankle of the leg.

(9) Wind Market(GB.31, Figure FA 1):
Located on the upper thigh. When you stand and erect with your hands stretching down along the side of your body, the tip of the middle-finger would reach a point onthe thigh. Five inches upward from the finger-tip point is Wind Market point, GB.31, as shown in Figure FA 1. This is one of the points to be used for treating Hemiplegia.

b. Needle To Be Used: On and a half inches in length.

c. Treatment: The patient lies flat and immobilized. You can give treatment to the above-mentioned Acupunctural points in this posture. Simply push the needle in, and, when it reaches the given depth, give several light stimuli or tappings by fingers before pulling it out. Since strong stimuli are not needed, the sensation of the needle is not to be felt. In the case of a patient experiencing constipation, give additional insertion to Gate Origin point, CV.4 in Figure FA 1(See Colitis).

d. Effects: When the ailment is not very serious, it is usually cured in two to four weeks after on treatment. When the ailment is very serious, it takes 20 to 25 weeks to be cured. (The following are the additional Acupunctural points to be used.)

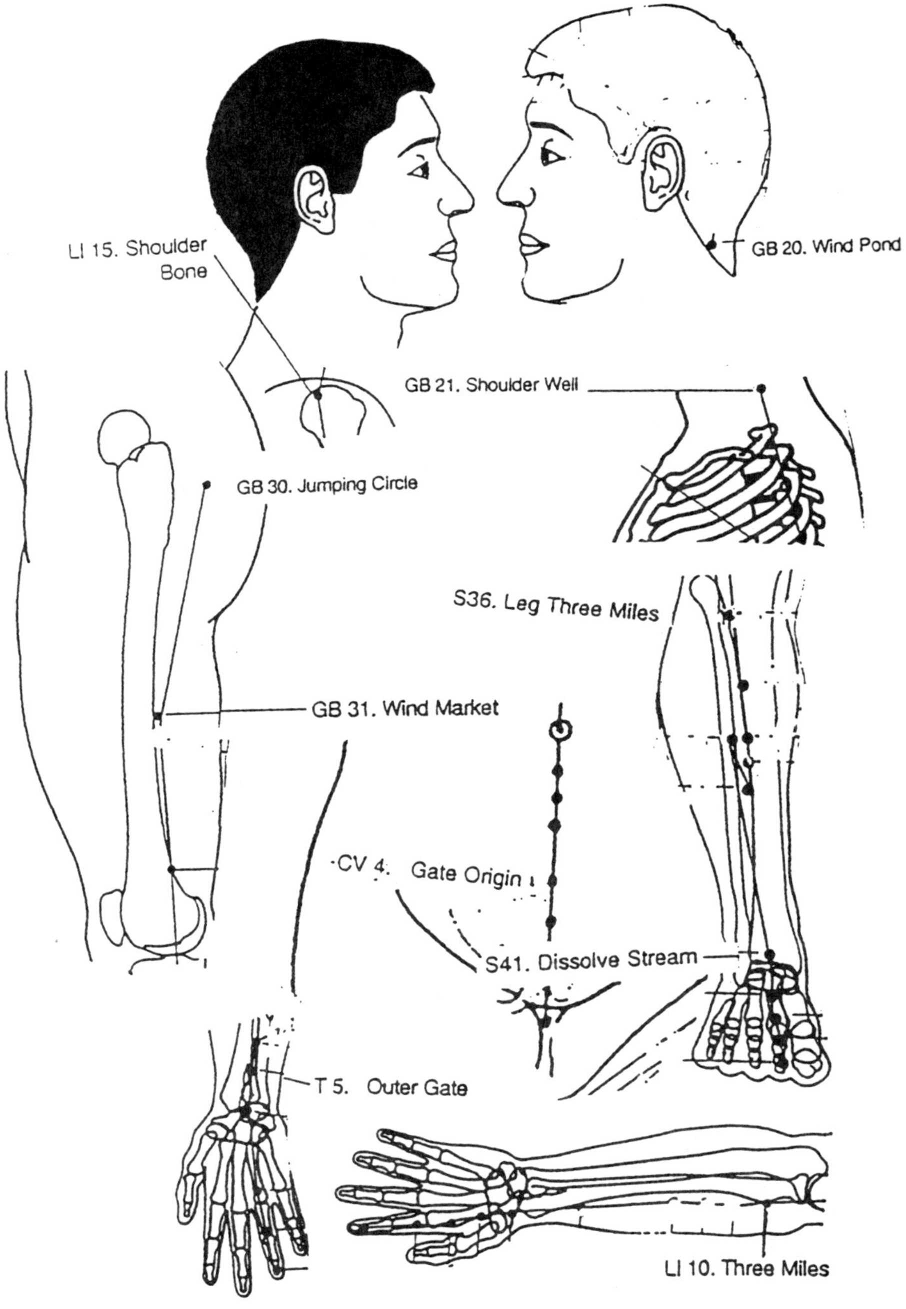
LI 15. Shoulder Bone
GB 20. Wind Pond
GB 21. Shoulder Well
GB 30. Jumping Circle
S36. Leg Three Miles
GB 31. Wind Market
CV 4. Gate Origin
S41. Dissolve Stream
T 5. Outer Gate
LI 10. Three Miles

FIGURE - FA1

HEMIPLEGIA(PART 2)

The following are the Acupuncture treatments for the paralyzed movements of one side of the body caused by after-effects of cerebral hemorrhage.

a. Shoulder Well(GB.21, Figure F 1):
The Acupuncture point, Shoulder Well, is at the midpoint of the shoulder. This point is effective for points in the shoulder, convulsion on the neck, neurasthenia, paralysis, etc. (From Chinese Acupuncture Handbook, P.114) Be sure that the insertion should not be too deep. A deep insertion may cause danger to the patient.

b. Wind Pond(B.10, Figure F 1):
See the section on Neurasthenia for explanation of this point. It is frequently used for treatment of Hemiplegia.

c. Shoulder Bone(LI.15, Figure F1)·
This point is located at the acromion process on each shoulder. Insertion may be made three-quarters of an inch to one full inch deep. This particular point treatment is made in the case of a patient feeling pain at the soulderjoints when he raises his arms upward along the back of the body. If the patient feels pain when he raises his arms in front of him, another point, Shoulder Well, is recommended for treatment.

d. Arm Three Miles(LI.10, Figure F1):
This point is at two inches down from the elbow joint on the exterior side of the radius.

e. Wind Market(GB.31, Figure F 1)
First you stand erect and stretch your hands down along the side of your body. Then the tip of the middle-finger reaches a certain part of the thigh. Five inches upward from the tip of the middle-finger is the Acupuncture point, called Wind Market.

f. Outer Gate(T.5, Figure F1)
This Acupuncture point is located at the back of the writst - two inches above the wrist-joint between the two arm-bones. When the needle reaches a certain depth (one-sixth of an inch), the patient experiences the feeling spreading from the shoulders and neck to the fingers. Give light stimulus for two or three minutes to the needle. Then, put the needle a bit deeper and give some more stimulus before pulling it out. This treatment is effective for such ailments as headaches, boothaches, pain in the chest, deafness, unconscousness, conspiration after child-delivery,etc.

g. Jumping Circle(GB.30, Figure F 1)
This Acupuncture point is located at each side of the hip. Have the patient lie on his side with the legs bent to 120 degree at the knee. Insert the needle straight down at the point, and, when the feeling reaches the affected parts, stop the insertion for three or four minutes. Then, put the needle one or two-tenths of an inch deeper and give some more stimulus for another three or four minutes before pulling the needle out.

The feeling reaches the affected parts, when the patient experiences a comfortable feeling. This treatment is effective for such ailments as lumbaraches,paraplegics,rheumatism, etc.

h. Leg Three Miles (S.36, Figure F 1)
See the Section on Neurasthenia.

i. Dissolve Stream(S.41, Figure F 1)
Located at the front side of the ankle. Use one-and-a-half an inch in depth.

j. Other Points Usually Used: GB.11, LI.4, GB.34, LV.3(See Figure F 1).

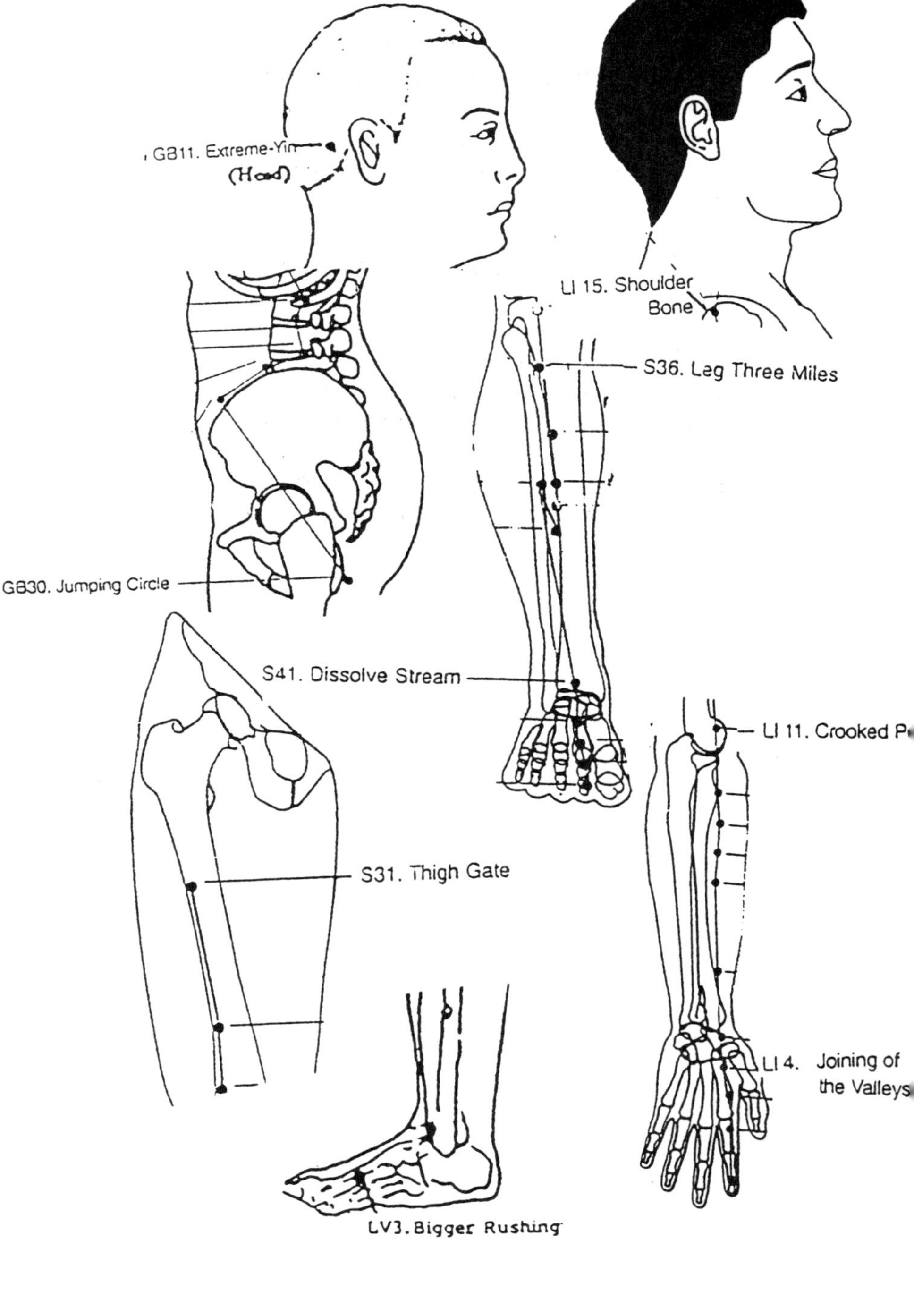
GB11. Extreme-Yin
(Head)
LI 15. Shoulder
Bone
S36. Leg Three Miles
GB30. Jumping Circle
S41. Dissolve Stream
LI 11. Crooked P
S31. Thigh Gate
LI 4. Joining of
the Valleys
LV3. Bigger Rushing

FIGURE-F1

2. HIGH BLOOD PRESSURE

The general symptoms of high blood pressure include heaviness of head, head-aches, buzzing in the ears, loss of memory, shortness of breath, feeling as if the abdomen is full, numbness of fingers, heaviness of limbs, etc. There are eight Acupuncture points for treatment of this ailment.

a. Anterior Summit(GV.20, Figure F 2)

Location: AT the top of head.
Needle: One and a half inches in length.
Depth of Insertion: One quarter of an inch.
Treatment: Have the patient sit upright, or let him lie on the side. Insert the needle up to the bone and give some stimulus or tappings before pulling it out.
Effects: This point is good for treatment of such ailments as paralysis,head-ache, dizziness, protcele,fever, nose blooding, deaf-mute,children's diarrhea,etc.

b. Heavenly Pillar(B.10, Figure F 2):
See treatment for Neurasthenia.

c. Heart Su (B.15, Figure F 2)

Location:Between the fifth and sixth thoracic vertebrae on each side.
Needle:One and a-half inch in length.
Depth of Insertion: One-half to three-fourths of an inch.
Treatment: Insert the needle to the proper depth, and providing stimulus for one minute before pulling it out.

Effective For: Such ailments as vomiting, epilepsy, fearfulness, and high blood-pressure.

d. Kidney Su(B.23, Figure F 2):

Location: Under the second lumbar vertebra on each side.
Needle: One-and a half inch in length.
Depth of Insertion: Three-quarters of an inch.
Treatment: Have the patient sit upright on the chair or lie flat on his stomach. The point is located at one and a half inch off to each side under the second lumbar vertebra. Insert the needle and commence some stimulus for one minute before pulling it out.

e. Man Welcome(S.9, Figure 2)

Location: On the front neck and on each side.
Needle: One and a half inch in length.
Depth of Insertion: Insert half an inch.
Treatment: Insert the needle up to the given depth and induce stimulation for one minute before extracting it. When the needle reaches the throat, change the needle-point outward so that the feeling may reach the head.

f. Water Division (CV.9, Figure F 2)

Location: One inch above the naval.
Needle: One and a half inch in length.
Depth of Insertion: Give some stimulus after having inserted the needle before pulling it out.

g. Inner Gate(P.6, Figure.F 2):

Location: Two inches above along the center-line from the wrist.
Needle: One and a half inch in length.
Depth of Insertion: One third to one half of an inch.
Treatment: Have the patient make a clenched fist which forces two bloodlines to surface on the arm above the writst. This point is located two inches above the wrist between the through twisting, the needle before exserted, some feeling should be felt at knees, shoulders, cheeks, or ears and down the middle-finger.
Effects: This treatment is good for such ailments as stomach-aches, vomitting, rib-pain, insomnia, colera, pains in the abdomen, etc.

h. Leq Three Miles(S.36, Figure F 2): See the Section on Neurasthenia.

i. Other Points Usually Treated:

Points B.10, K.25, and P.4(See Figure F 2) are also favorably use for treating high bolld-pressure. To ease the blood-pressure to the lowest point, the point K 25, located on the left side of the body, is considered most effective. High blood-pressure may be eased by one treatment or by as many as ten treatments depending upon the severity and sensitivity of the ailment.

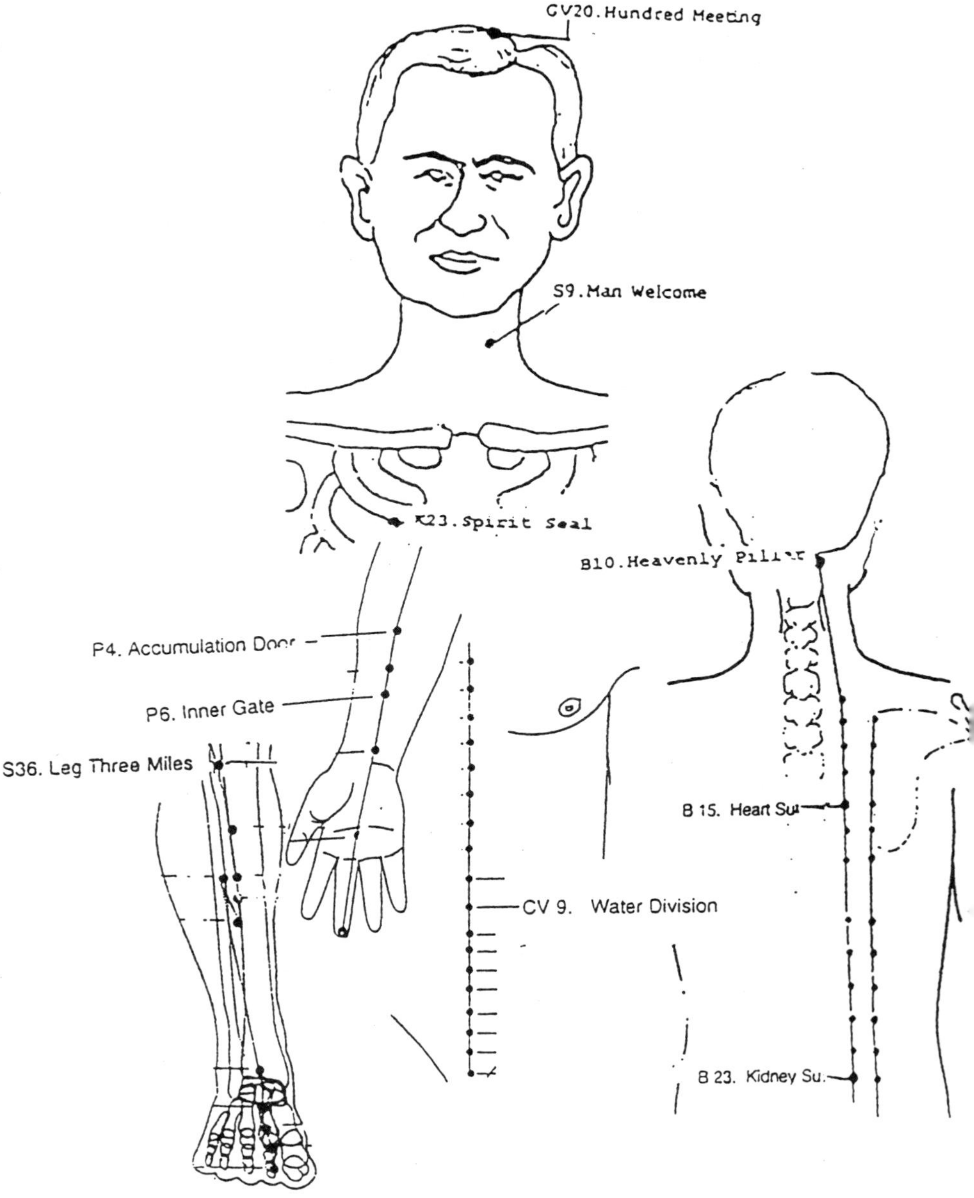
GV20. Hundred Meeting
S9. Man Welcome
K23. Spirit Seal
B10. Heavenly Pillar
P4. Accumulation Door
P6. Inner Gate
S36. Leg Three Miles
B 15. Heart Su
CV 9. Water Division
B 23. Kidney Su.

FIGURE - F2

3. INFLUENZA AND COLD

Cold is an ailment that may occur at any time throughout the year. When the temperature changes due to the changing seasons, we are likely to catch cold of some kind. The symptoms include coldness, fever, headache, cough, sneezing, snivelling, stuffy nose, weariness and feebleness at limbs, soreness at throat, etc.

a. Wind Gate(B.12, Figure F 3):
See the Section on Neurasthenia.
Location: Wind Gate is located at the first thoracic vertebra.

b. Joining of the Valley(LI.4, Figure F3):
Location: This point is located between the first and the second fingers.
Needle: One and a half inch in length.
Depth of insertion: One third to one half on an inch.
Treatment: Insert the proper needle by twisting it slowly. Leave the needle at the point for thirty minutes or so, and , then, pulls it out quickly. This point, Joining of the Valley, should be used for a pregnant woman. When the patient feels headache, another needle may be inserted at the point, Eye Bone(See Figure F 3). If the headache remains severe, either one of the following points may be used for additional insertion: Head Tied and Yulkyul (See Figure F 3). For the ailment of coughs, use these two points, Foot Marsh(L.5) and Lung Su(B.13). For stuffy nose, use the point, Yung-yang. When the patient feels dull and

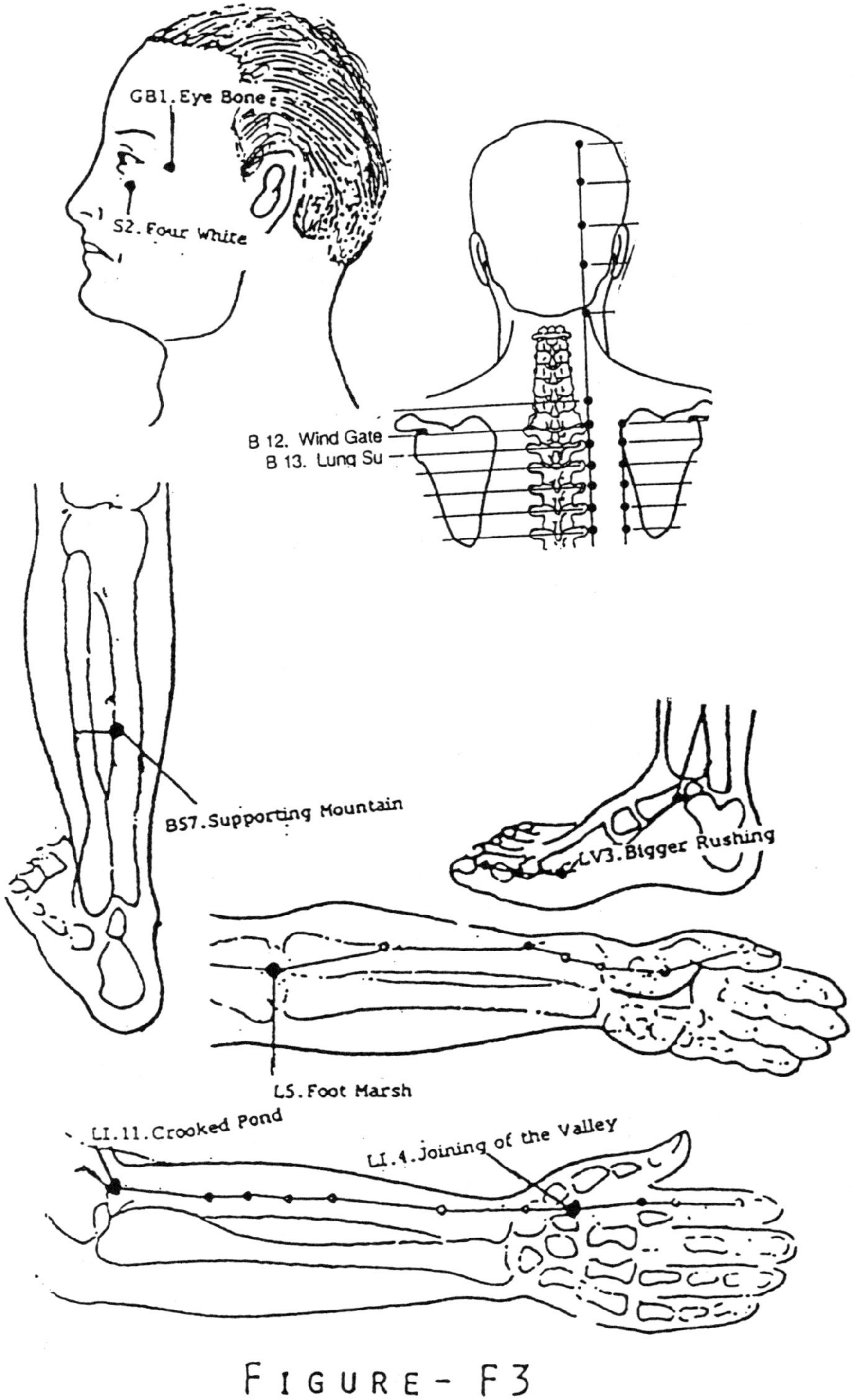
GB1. Eye Bone
S2. Four White
B 12. Wind Gate
B 13. Lung Su
B57. Supporting Mountain
LV3. Bigger Rushing
L5. Foot Marsh
LI. 11. Crooked Pond
LI. 4. Joining of the Valley

FIGURE- F3

aches all over the body, including limbs, use the points, Crooked Pond(LI.11) and Supporting Mountain(B.57). Also use the points, Eye Bone (GB.1) and Four White(S.2). See Figure F 3 for the above mentioned points.

4. EPILEPTIC FITS

Strong emotional shocks or angry rage can cause a person to lose consciousness, accompanied by such symptoms as convulsions of the whole body, foaming at the mouth, and grinding of teeth. This kind of fit may last from minutes to hours depending upon its severeness. Acupunctural points to be used: See Figure 4 in the following page.

a. Joining of the Valley (LI.4,Figure F 4): Located between the first and the second fingers.

b. Bigger Pushing (LV.3, Figure F 4): Located between the first and the second metatarsal bones of the foot.

c. Other Points Usually Treated:

CV.12;CV.9; B.8 (or B.20);B.2;B.10; GV.20;GV.12;
and B.7 in Figure F 4.

Needles To Be Used: One and one third inches in length.
Depth of Insertion: One third to two fifths of and inch.
Treatment: In the case of a patient with the symptoms of losing consciousness and falling down, one may insert the needle with strong stimulus at the given depth, and provide additional stimulus before pulling the needle

out. One may preferably put two needles into the points, Joining of the Valley(LI.4, Figure F 4), and give stimulus alternately to each needle. If the ailment is not too serious, the patient may wake up immediately and gain consciousness by the Joining of the Valley insertion alone. When insertions at the two Joining of the Valley points are not enough to awake the patient, then insert additional needles at the Bigger Pushing(LV 3, Figure $)in the similar fashion. When four insertions were made on hands and feet, the patient would surely wake up. If the fit is very strong, the patient may again lose consciousness after having been awakened once. If this is the case, one may insert the needles at Bigger Pushing on each foot while giving strong stimulus to the needles.

Effects: One treatment should be enough. The epileptic fits are distinguished from other similar ailments by feeling the pulse and breathing, which are supposed to be normal but a bit weaker.

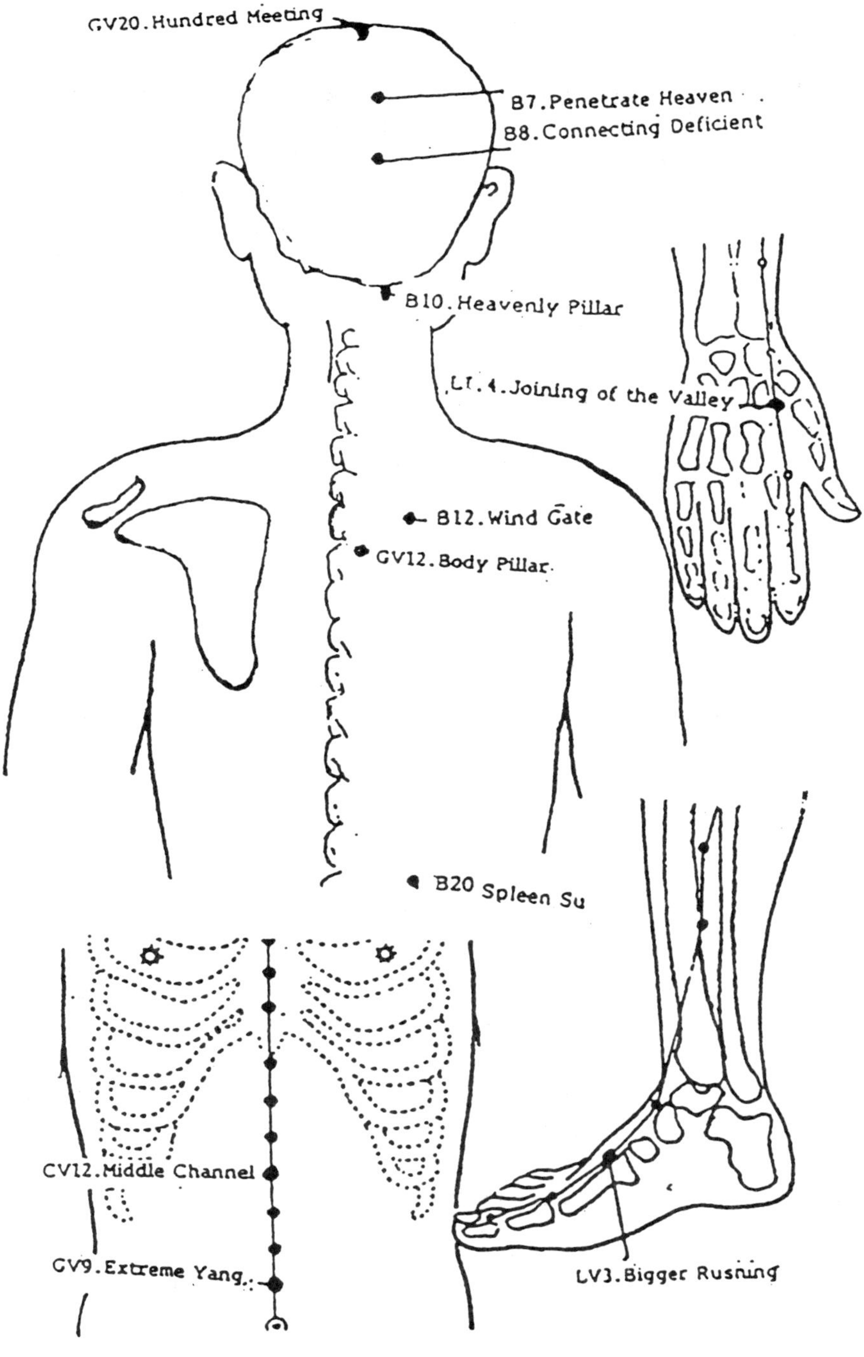
GV20. Hundred Meeting
B7. Penetrate Heaven
B8. Connecting Deficient
B10. Heavenly Pillar
LI. 4. Joining of the Valley
B12. Wind Gate
GV12. Body Pillar
B20 Spleen Su
CV12. Middle Channel
GV9. Extreme Yang
LV3. Bigger Rushing

FIGURE - F4

5. NEURASTHENIA

The characteristic symptoms of Neurasthenia include dizziness, dullness of the brain, headaches, disturbances in dreams, fatigue, weariness, feebleness, etc. These symptoms vary for different individuals and by the duration of the ailment. Five Acupunctural points may be utilized for treatment. (See Figure F 5):

a. Heavenly Pillar (B.10, Figure 5):

Location: This point is located between the first and the second cervical vertebrae under the Occipital bone on each side.
Needle: An one and a half inch needle should be employed.
Depth of Insertion: When the ailment is very serious, the patient may be overly sensitive, so that the needle of an inch in depth should be adequate. If the ailment is not so serious, the needle should be put a bit deeper—three fourths of an inch.
Treatment: It is recommended that the patient sits on the chair with his hands folded on the table and his head resting on the hands. Insert the needle straight down to the given depth, and provide some light stimulus to the needle. It is not necessary to provide any strong stimulus that might reach certain other areas of the body. Slow and tender tapping of the needle causes a comfortable feeling.
Effects: The treatment of this point is very effective for those patients who are unable to sleep at night or who are overly conscious of slightest

noise, which might disturb the patient in dreams.

b. Wind Pond(GB.20, Figure F 5)

Location: This point is located between the Trapezius and Sternocleidomastoid under the Occipital bone on each side.
Needle: One and a half inch in length.
Depth of insertion: Three quarters of an inch.
Treatment: Have the patient sit on the chair with his hands on the table and his head resting on his hands. When the needle is inserted into the left point, the needle point would be aimed toward the right eye, and, when the needle is inserted into the right point, the needle point would be aimed toward the left eye. Provide some tapping stimulus to the needle for twenty seconds in every minute for the duration of five minutes. The resonance of the stimulated needle should be felt in the patient's head around the eye and also around the shoulder. such a resonance would provide a comfortable feeling to the patient.
Effects: This treatment is effective for easing such ailments as headache, cold, fever, cough, toothache,whooping cough, and ear diseases.

c. Lung Su (B.13, Figure F 5):

Location: Lung Su is located on the back --one and a half inch below the third thoracic vertebra on each side.

Needle: One and a half inches in length.

Depth of Insertion: About one inch.

Treatment: Have the patient sit up right on the chair or lie flat on his stomach. Insert the needle up to the given depth, and provide some moderate stimulus to the needle for two minutes before extracting the needle. Let the patient have deep breathing for a few times.

Effects: This treatment is effective for easing such ailments as cough and whooping-cough.

d. Great Shrine(CV.14, Figure F 5):

Location: Located at a little below the Xiphoid process.

Needle: One and a half inch in length.

Treatment: Have the patient lie on his back with his head resting on a pillow. Insert the needle slowly to the given depth, and give some stimulus to the needle for one minute before pulling it out.

Effects: Acupunctural treatment on this point is effective for relieving mental disorders, fearfulness, pleurisy, stomachaches,etc.

e. Leg Three Miles (S.36, Figure F 5)

Location: Under the knees, slightly to exterior,between tibia and fibula.

Needle: One and a half inch in length.

Depth of Insertion: One half to one inch.

Treatment: The patient feels dull traction at the point, and it spreads to the leg and, sometimes, to the abdomen.

Effects: This point is effective for such

ailments as dizziness, stomachaches, vomiting, diarrhea, constipation, toothaches, etc. Insomnia, disturbing dreams, and lack of appetite can be cured by one or more treatments, as mentioned earlier. It is possible that the other symptoms can also be cured by ten or more treatments.

Insertions can be made very effectively at the points which are quite sensitive to finger-pressure.

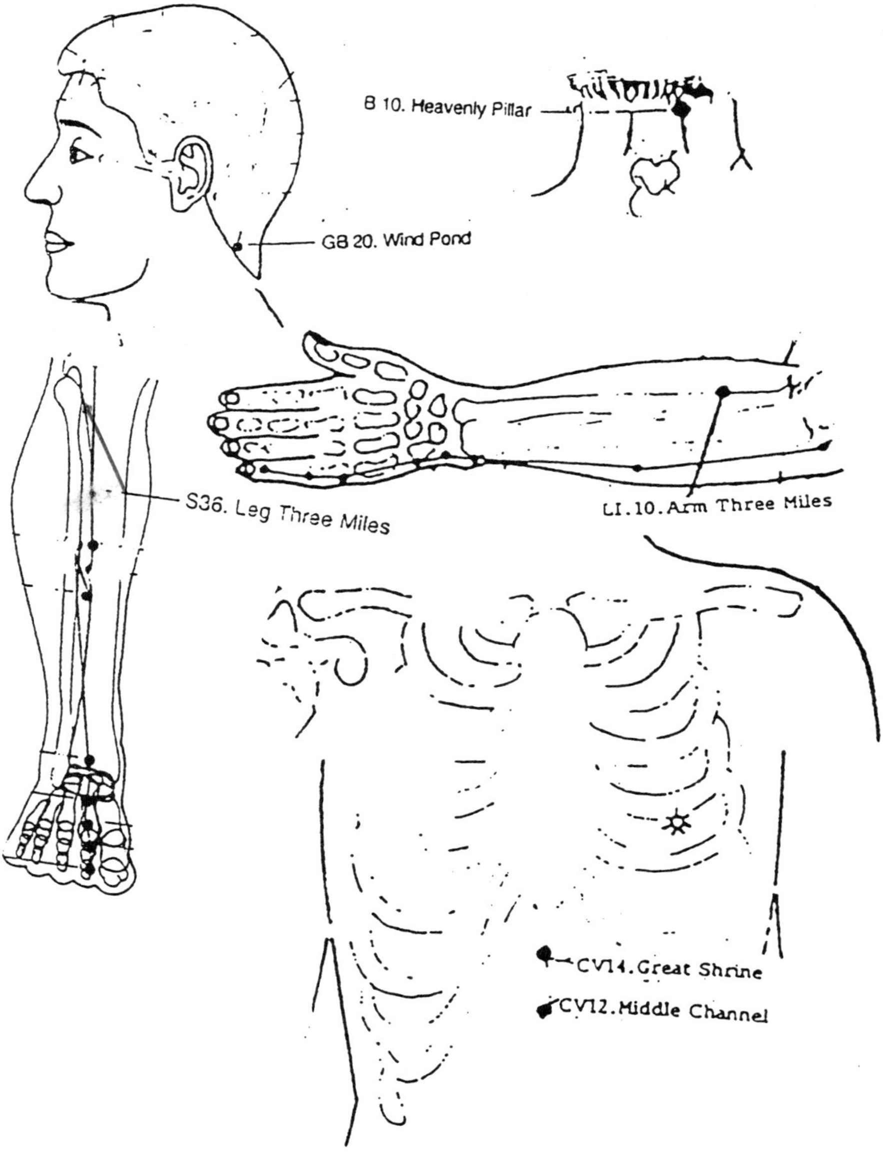
B 10. Heavenly Pillar
GB 20. Wind Pond
S36. Leg Three Miles
LI.10. Arm Three Miles
CV14. Great Shrine
CV12. Middle Channel

FIGURE- F5

6. INDIGESTION FROM DRINKING

Stomach may swell due to excessive drinking of alcoholic beverages. The Patient is likely to have pain in the stomach and he may vomit. The patient may feel relieved of the pain through repetitive drinking. The relevant Acupuncture points are shown in Figure F 39.

a. Middle Channel CV.12 (Figure F 39)

b. Arm Three Miles LI.10 (Figure F 39)

Depth of Insertion: At the point CV.12, one and a half inch is adequate, whereas at the point LI.10, one inch is recommended. It is better to give strong tapping stimulation to the needle at both points. It is most likely that the patient might have his liver damaged by excessive alcoholic drinking. The above- mentioned treatment is quite effective in helping the damaged liver to recover to its normal state. When the affected liver is restored to its normal state, it makes easier for the patient to stop drinking.

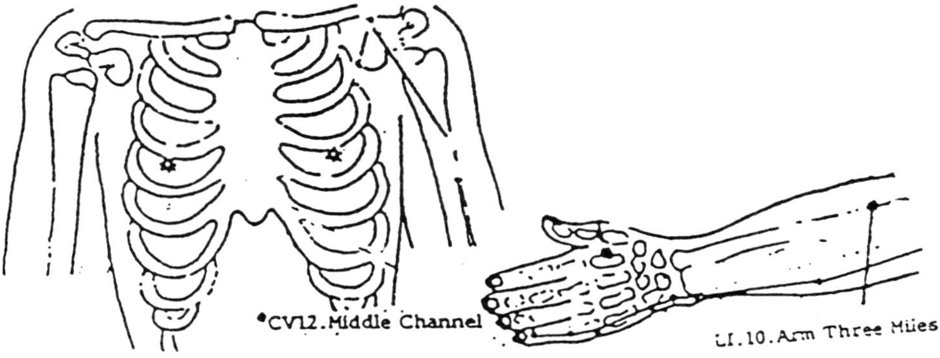

FIGURE- F39

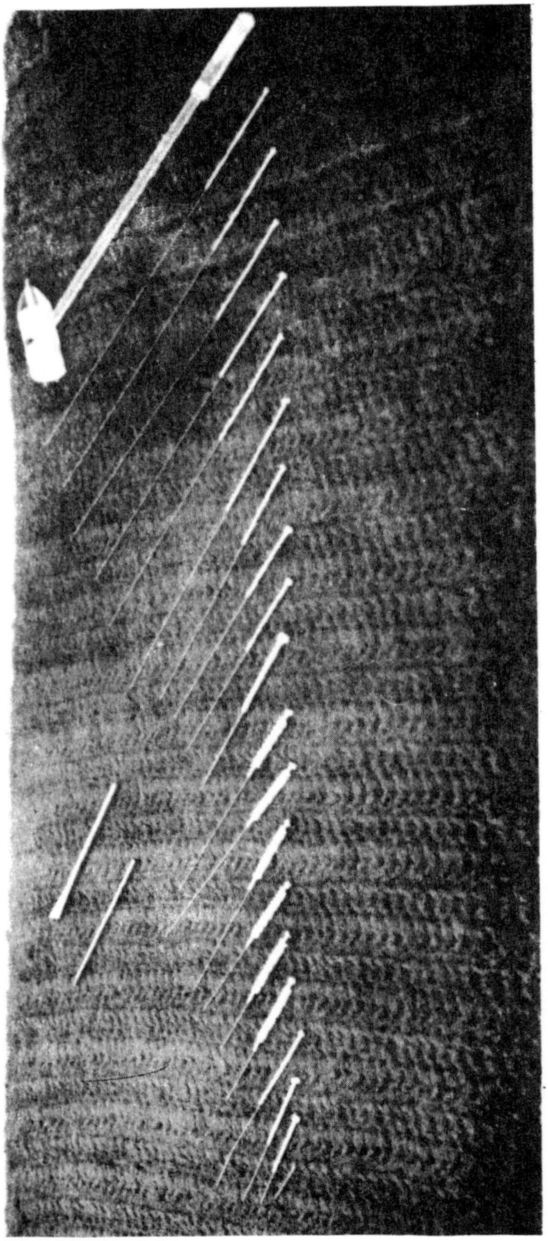

ACUPUNCTURE NEEDLES

CHAPTER II

MALFUNCTIONING OF THE ARMS

CHAPTER II
MALFUNCTIONING OF THE ARMS

1. CARPAL BONES

When the wrist swells and aches, causing uneasy or restricted movement of the hands, the outer side of the wrist usually gets swollen and aches rather than the interior side.

For treatment, the point T5.Outer Gate in Figure F 6 is usually utilized.

Needle: One and a half inch in length.
Depth of Insertion: About half an inch.
Treatment: Have the patient sit upright or lie flat and let his hands rest on the knee of the Acupuncturist. Press the needle into the skin vertically until it reaches the given depth, so that its feeling gets to the affected area. Give a tapping stimulus to the needle for two or tree minutes: thereupon, push the needle a little deeper. Again, give a tapping stimulus for two or tree minutes before pulling the needle out. In the case of acute arthritis, which causes sever pain, seven or eight needles may be inserted into the skin at the point T4.Yang Pond(See Figure F.6) and the immediate area around it with the depth of one tenth or two fifths of an inch.
Effects: Acute arthritis can be eased by giving a treatment every day for two or three days. Chronic ailments can be cured by five or six treatments--giving one treatment every other day.

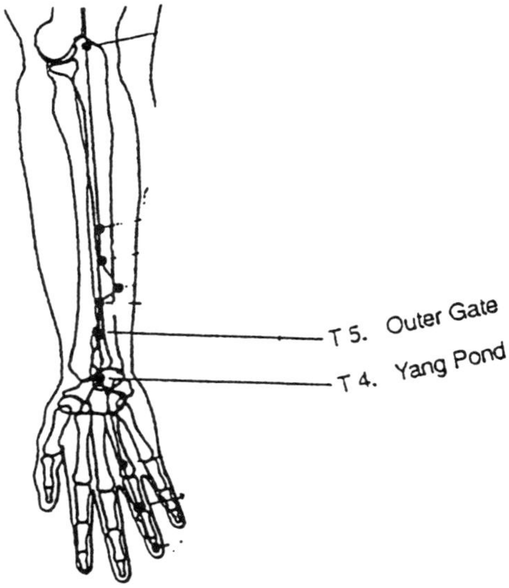

FIGURE-F6

2. NEURALGIA IN THE UPPER ARM

The patient may feel pains or discomfort (such as being strained, sore , heavy, or irritated) from the upper arms through the arm-joints down to the thumb. Two insertion points, GB21.Shoulder Well and T12.Thawing Luo River in Figure F.7 are recommended for the treatment. The location of the point GB.21 and how to insert the needle are explained under the Section - Pains in the Shoulder.

The point T12.Thawing Luo River is located at the center of the exterior side of the upper arm. The depth of insertion should be one half to three fifths of an inch. Have the patient sit erect or lie down side-way, and insert the needle at the point vertically with slight tapping. When the needle gets to the prescribed depth and the feeling of its effect reaches from the elbow to the thumb along the channel of pain, stop the needle at that level and give a tapping stimulation to the needle for two or three minutes before pulling it slowly out. The tapping stimulus gives the patient a comfortable feeling. Any stronger stimulation should preferably be avoided because it may cause a shock similar to electric current.

Effects: One or two treatments are sufficient for those patients having been afflicted with the ailment for only a few weeks. For those who have had the ailment for more than a month, it is necessary for them to receive the treatment on every other day for five to seven days. For those patient who have had the ailment for more than a year, at least ten treatments are required.

Other Points Usually Employed:GV13.Kiln Path,B10.HeavenlyPillar,B11.BigShuttle,SI.10. ShoulderBlade,LI.11.Crooked Pond,LI.10.Arm Three Miles,etc.,in Figure F.7.

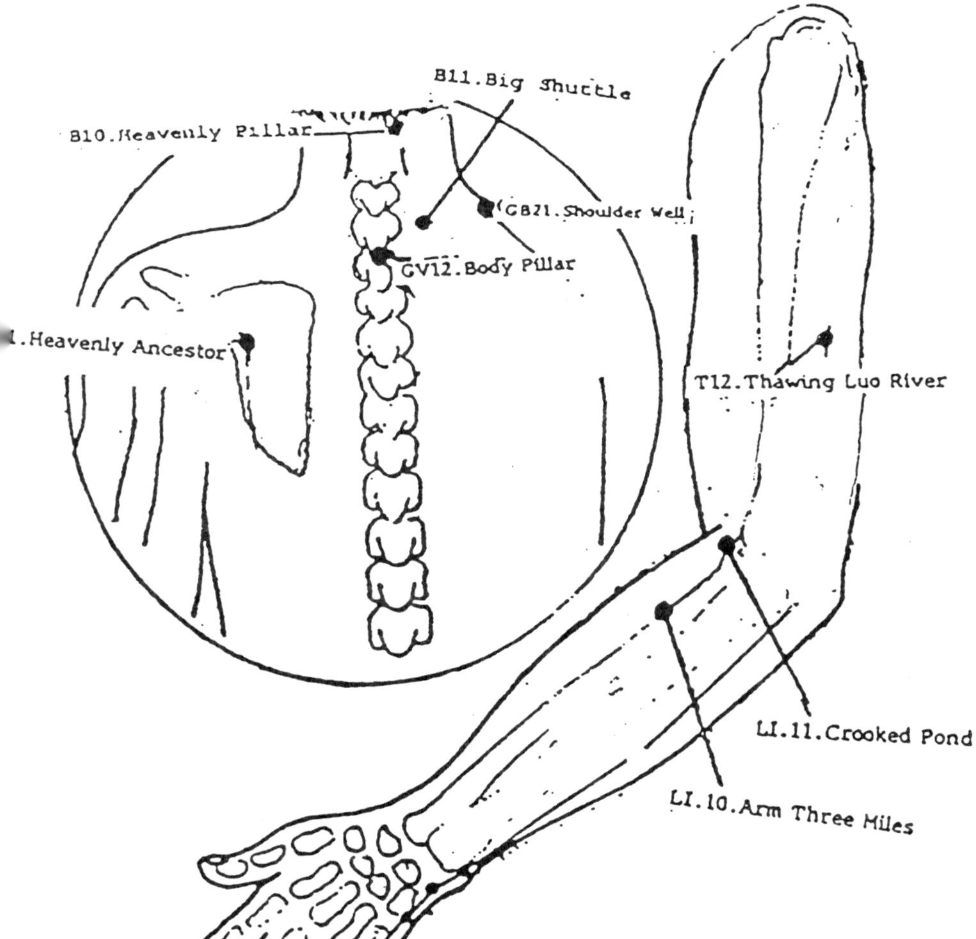
B11.Big Shuttle
B10.Heavenly Pillar
GB21.Shoulder Well
GV12.Body Pillar
.Heavenly Ancestor
T12.Thawing Luo River
LI.11.Crooked Pond
LI.10.Arm Three Miles

FIGURE- F 7

3. PAINS IN THE CARPAL BONES

The symptoms; the patient is unable to bend his hands, because it is very painful at the wrist-joints; and the movement of the thumb also cause much pain in most cases.

Acupunctural points to be used, as shown in Figure F.8.

a. LI.6.Inclined Passage, Figure F.8

   This point is located at two inches above the wrist.

b. SI.11, LI.10.,P4,P7,T4,etc.,in Figure F.8.

   One can feel a small muscle covering the radius bone. Below the muscle one feels a little hollow point. If you pressed the point with your finger, you may feel throbbing spreading toward the thumb.

   The depth of insertion at this point is one their to one half of an inch.

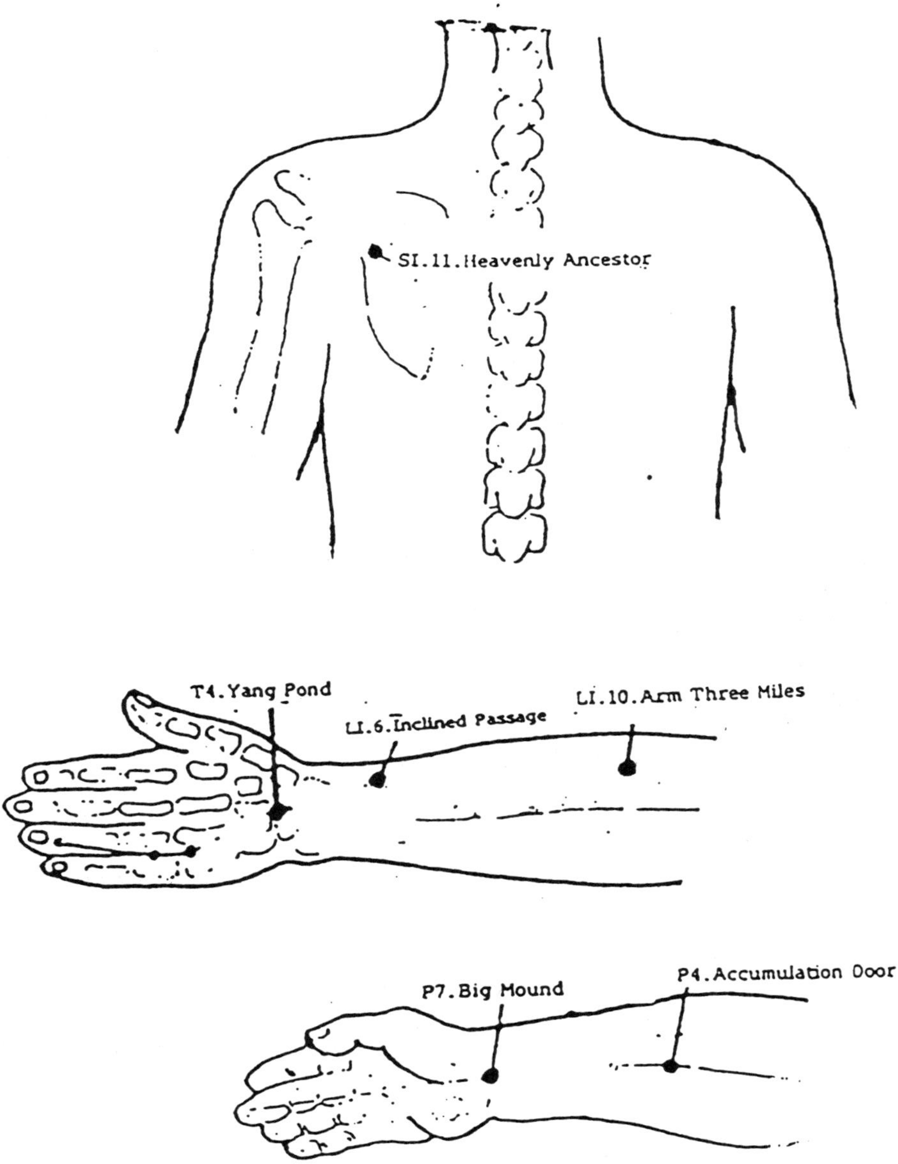
SI.11.Heavenly Ancestor
T4.Yang Pond
LI.6.Inclined Passage
LI.10.Arm Three Miles
P7.Big Mound
P4.Accumulation Door

FIGURE- F8

4. SCAPULA

When the patient lifts his hands or moves them around, he feels pain at the shoulder joints. Depending upon where the pain is felt, two different Acupunctural points are employed for the treatment. If the pain is felt at the rear deltoid-muscle, whenever the patient moves or raises his hands upward, the needle would be inserted at GB.21.Shoulder Well in Figure F.9. If the pain is felt at the front lower portion of the deltoid-muscle, whenever the patient moves or raises his hands backward, the needle should be inserted at the point LI.16.Great Bone or LI.15.Shoulder Bone, as shown in Figure F.9. And additional insertion at the point SI.12.Facing the Wind may be made simultaneously along with either of the above-mentioned two insertions for more effective treatment.
Acupuncture points to be used, as shown in Figure F.9:

a. GB.21.Shoulder Well: Located at the rear of the shoulder two inches below the arm-pit under acromion process.

b. LI.16.Great Bone: Located between the point of clavicle and acromion process.

c. LI.15.Shoulder Bone: Located at the end of acromion process where humerus joints.

d. SI.12.Facing the Wind.

e. GV.13.,LI.11,L1,L4,and L6:These points are also employed.

Needle To Be Used: One and one half inches in length.

<u>Depth of Insertion</u>: Three quarters to four fifths of an inch for all the above points.

<u>Treatment</u>: Have the patient sit upright or lie on his side with the aching side up and his arm bent toward his chest. At GB21. <u>Shoulder Well</u>,point the needle outward and upward and insert it by slight tapping. When the needle reaches the given depth and its feeling gets to the aching part of the shoulder joints, give some stimulation to the needle for a few moments in such a way that the needle point touches the muscle. Again, give some tapping to the needle for a few seconds, and then insert the needle a bit deeper in order to provide its feeling to the desired parts. The tapping stimulation helps the patient with a comfortable feeling, but if the stimulation is too strong so that the patient cannot bear it, we must withdraw slightly the needle by making it less deep and repeat the above procedures. The insertion at LI.16.<u>Great Bone</u> may be made in the same manner as in the case of GB.21.<u>Shoulder Well</u>. It must be emphasized that the effect of the needle insertion should be felt in the entire area of shoulder joints. The similar procedures are involved in regard to LI.15.<u>Great Bone</u>;the feeling of the needle should be directed toward the deltoid. At SI.12.<u>Facing the Wind</u>, one may insert the needle in the same manner as described in the above.

<u>Effects</u>: The ailments of less than six months can be cured through a period of seven to ten separate treatments. Shoulder pains, which are caused by excessive bodily exertion, can be more easily cured, but the ailments caused by external wounds are so stubborn and persistent that any quick recovery may not be easily anticipated.

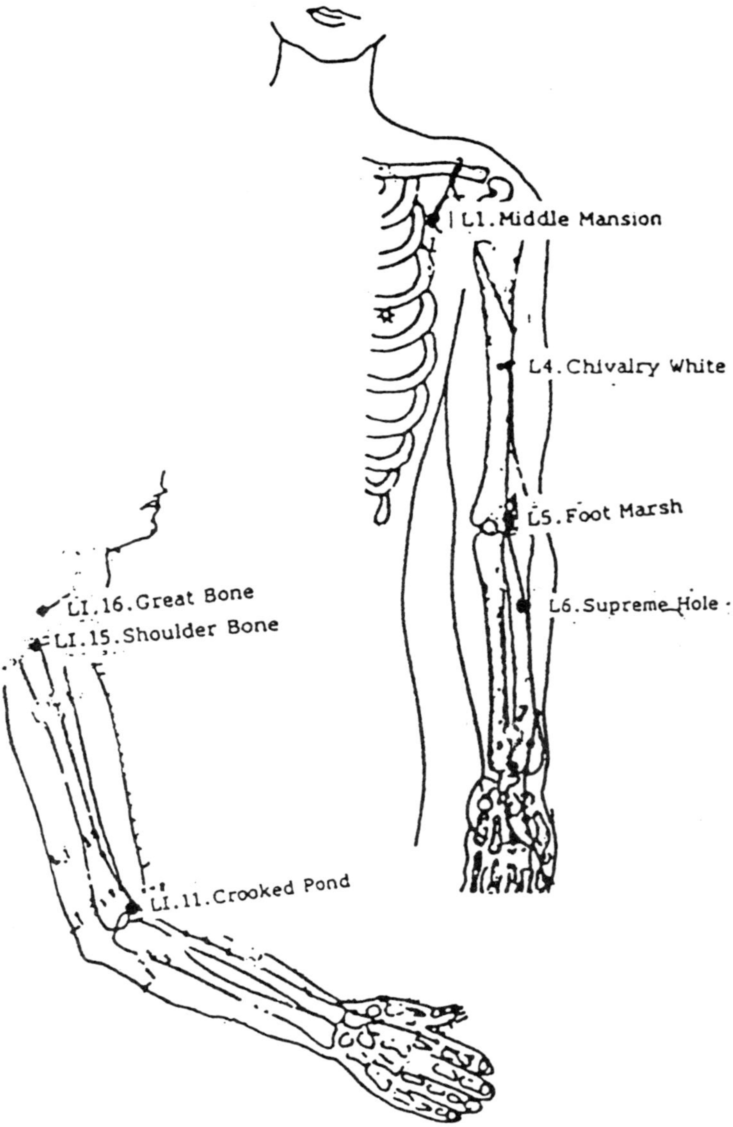
L1. Middle Mansion
L4. Chivalry White
L5. Foot Marsh
L6. Supreme Hole
LI. 16. Great Bone
LI. 15. Shoulder Bone
LI. 11. Crooked Pond

FIGURE-F9

5. PAINS IN THE HANDS

The patient feels acute pain and numbness on the palm and fingers. He may find his hands impossible to move about when he gets up in the morning. Two Acupuncture points can be employed for the treatment:P4.Accumulation Door and P5.The Intermediary in Figure F.10.

P4.Accumulation is located at the point about five inches above the wrist joint, while P5.The Intermediary is located at the point three inches above the wrist joint. One can feel the two tendons, and The Intermediary is located between them, as shown in Figure F.10.

Depth of Insertion:For the treatment at the point P4, the depth should be three quarters or four fifths of an inch, and for that at the point P5 should be half an inch or a bit deeper.

Treatment: Have the patient lie flat on his back and ask him how painful he feels while holding his ailing hands. If the pain is severe, choose the point P4, but if the pain is relatively mild, choose the point P5.

Insert the needle vertically with slight tapping. When the needle reaches the prescribed depth and its feeling gets to the center of the patient's alm, where the pain is felt, stop any further insertion. Provide light tappings to the needle for two or three minutes, insert the needle one tenth of an inch deeper, and repeat the light tapppings for another two or three minutes before extracting the needle.

If one treatment is not sufficient to alleviate the pain, then repeat the above procedures two or three more times. If the pain appears to be reduced at first one or two treatments, one should try to press for the needle feeling.

Effects: If the ailment has not developed to an advanced stage, it can be cured by two or three days' treatments -- only one treatment per day. If its has persisted, then provide five or six days' continous treatments.

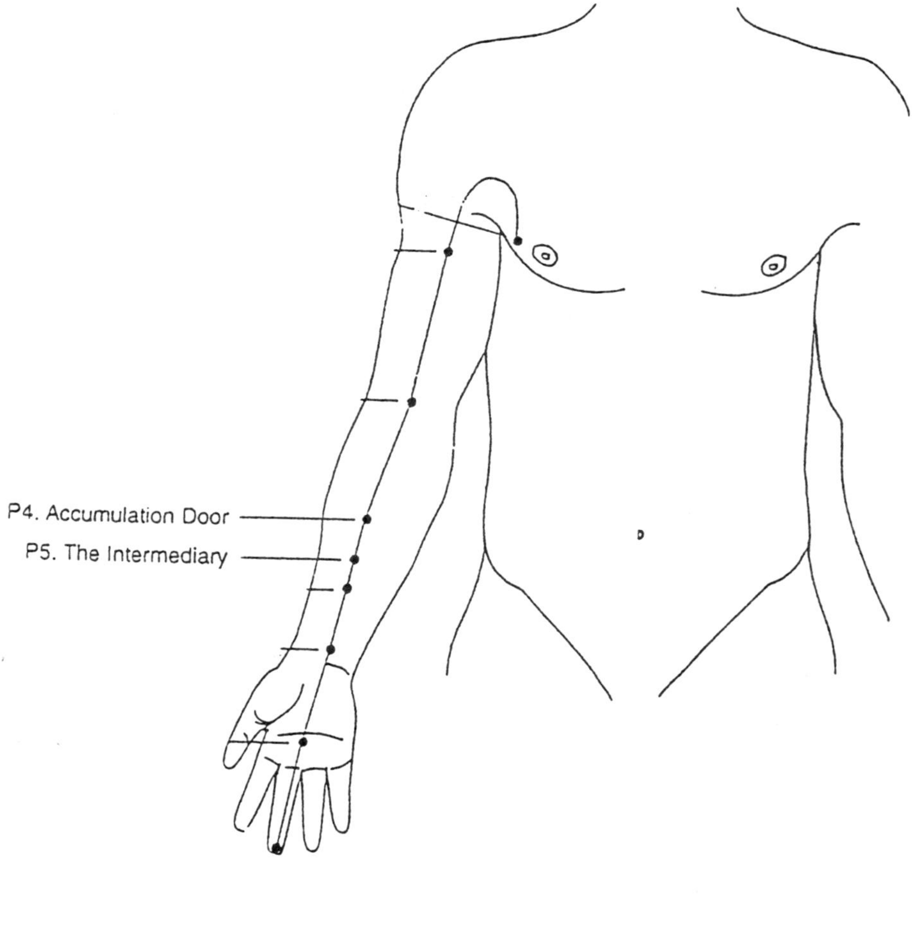

FIGURE- F10

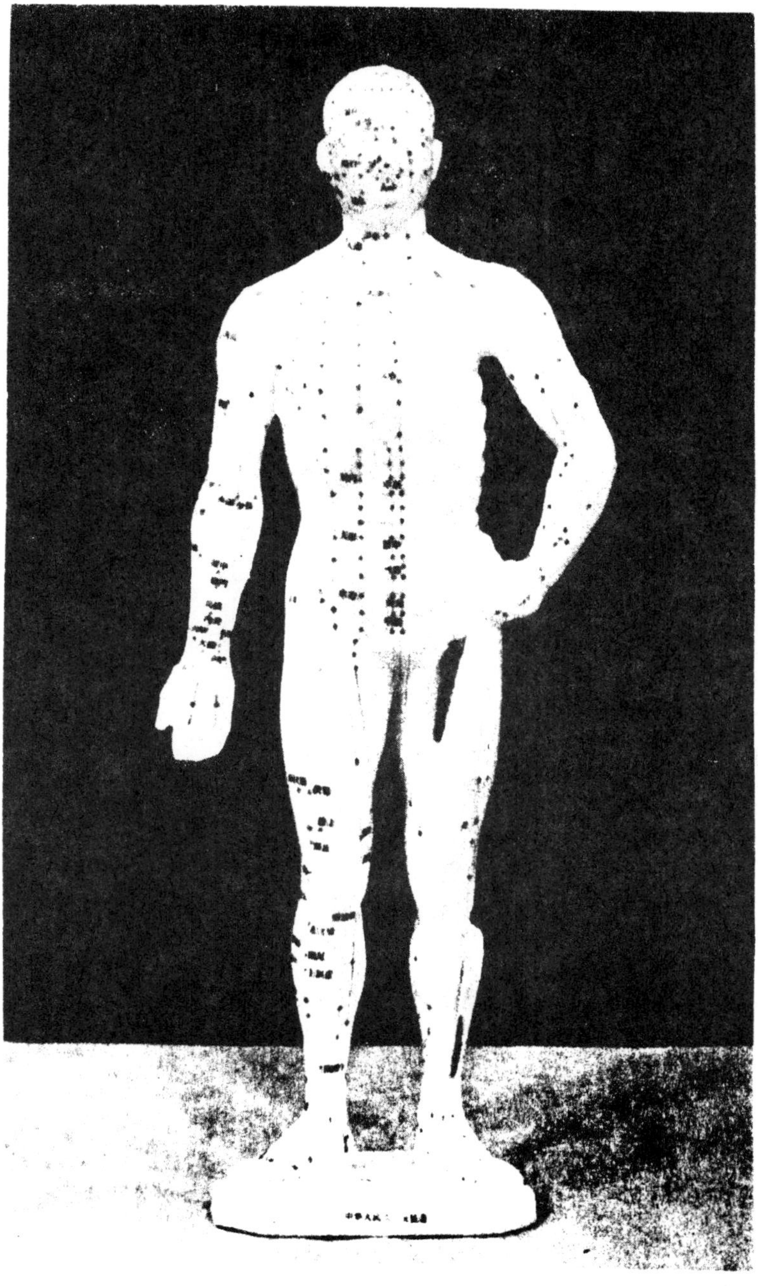

- FRONT -

PICTURE SHOWING MERIDIANS AND ACUPUNCTURE POINTS

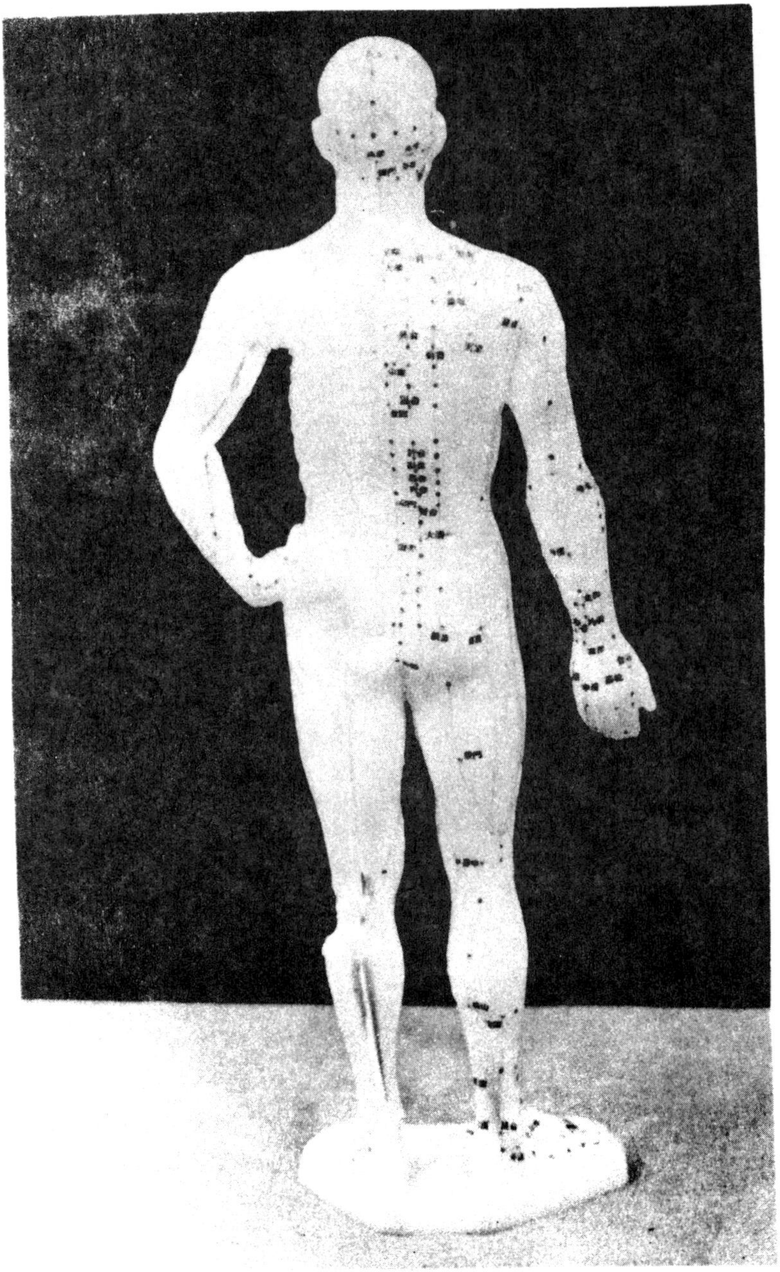

- BACK -

PICTURE SHOWING MERIDIANS AND ACUPUNCTURE POINTS

CHAPTER III

AILMENTS IN THE CHEST

CHAPTER III
AILMENTS IN THE CHEST

1. COUGHS

Here the cough means the chronic bronchial catarrh.

The recommended Acupunctural point CV.22.Heaven Rushing is shown in Figure F.11.

Location: The point is found at the upper end of the sternum between the larynx and the bronchus, where if pressed with finger it causes coughs. This is the most sensitive point for coughing.

Depth of Insertion: One half to three fifths of an inch.

Treatment: Have the patient sit upright, and the acupuncturist takes a position at his right side. First, insert the needle up to a third of the prescribed depth and provide some stimulation for one or two minutes. Then, put some pressure to the needle end, but make sure that the needle remains steady at the same depth. At this point, should the patient feel like coughing, he must communicate it by signal. Pull the needle up to the skin level. Wait until the impulse to cough subsides, and then push the needle back to the prescribed depth. Repeat the above treatment for a period of two or three times.

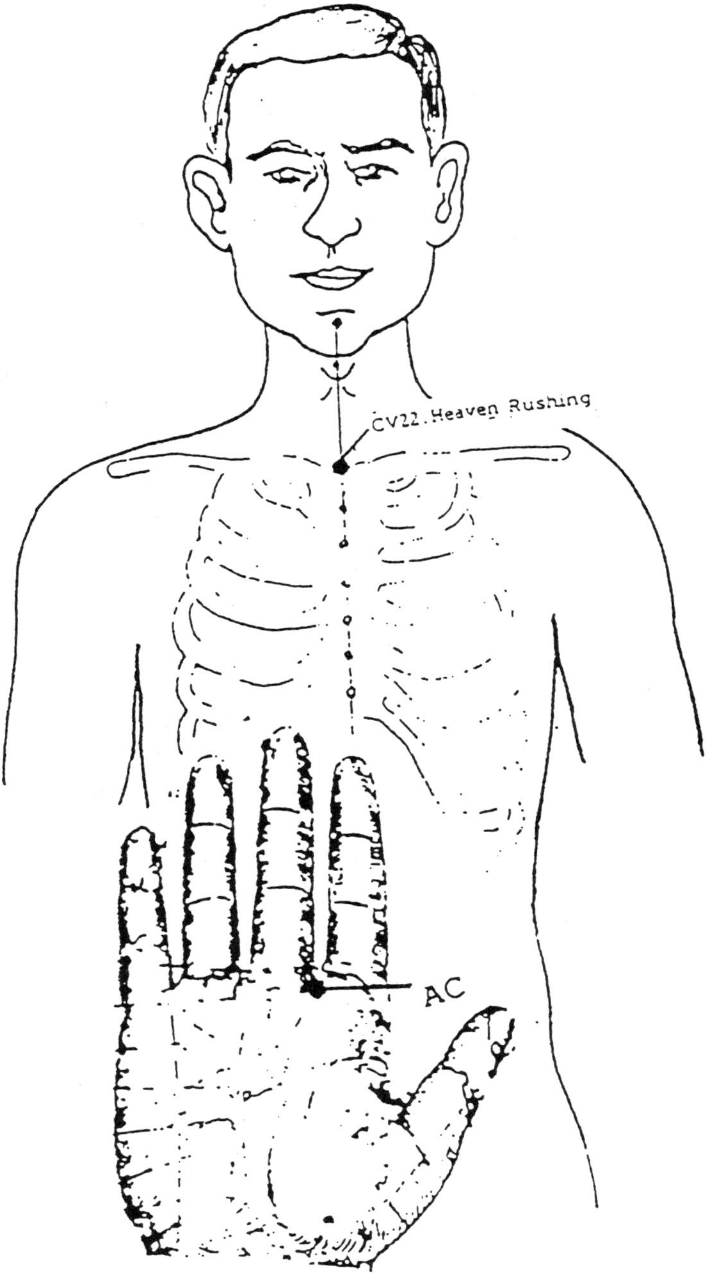

FIGURE- F11

2. SHORT BREATH

The patient experiences a difficulty of deep breathing, and he may often feel cocking from the chest.

The recommended Acupunctural points, B13.Lung Su and CV.20.Splendor Covering are shown in Figure F.12.

Location: These points are located at the sternum between the first and second ribs.

Depth of Insertion: One to one and half inches.

Treatment: In the case of the point CV.20,when the needle reaches the prescribed depth, provide light stimulation (almost touching the bone) for two minutes before pulling the needle out. The patient would feel the sensation of pleasure at this point.

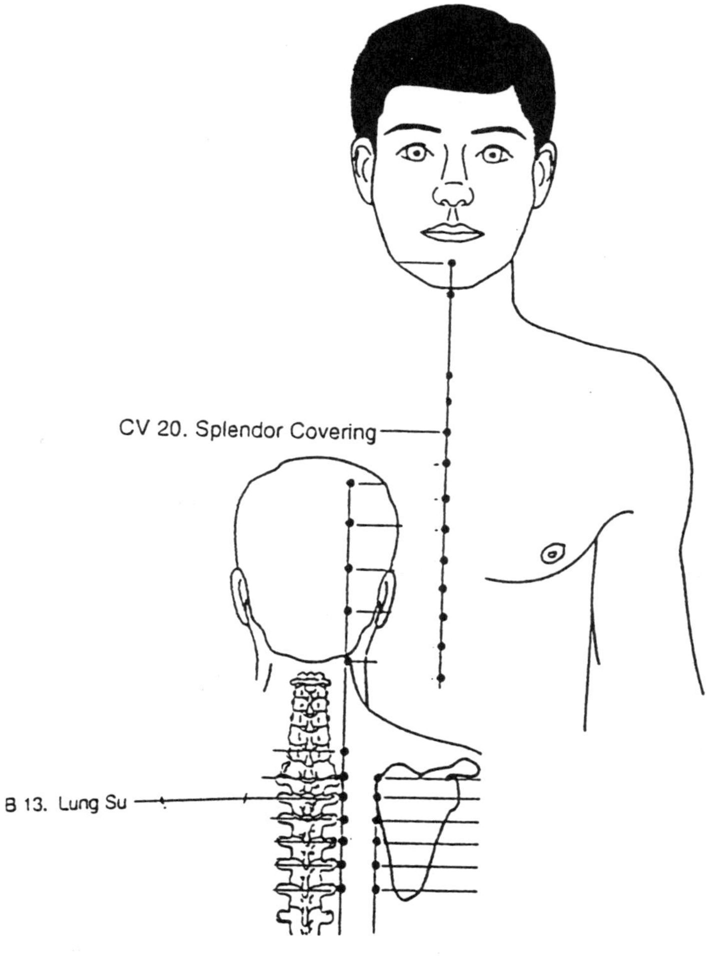

FIGURE-F12

3. BRONCHIAL ASTHMA

The patient shows such symptoms as gurgling in the throat, coughing, short breath, or heaviness in the chest.

The following are the utilized Acupunctural points, as illustrated in Figure F.13.

a. B13.Lung Su: Located under the third thoracic vertebra, half an inch off to each side of the back.

b. CV.22.Heaven Rushing:See the Section on "Cough".

c. S11.Qi Shelter:Located at the lower end of sternocleidomastoid on each side.

d. K26.Admist Elegance: Located under the alongside the sternum.

Depth of Insertion:

Point B13: Three to three and half inches.
Point CV.22:One half to three and half inches.
Point S11: One third to two fifths of an inch.
Point K26: Three fifths to four fifths of an inch.

Treatment: The patient should be in a sitting position. For the treatment of point B13:when the needle is inserted into the proper depth, provided moderate stimulation for two minutes before extracting the needle. Then,let the patient exercise deep breathing for a few moments. For the treatment of point CV.22,see the section on "cough". As to the treatment of point S11, point the needle end downward and innerward. When the resonance of the needle reaches into the chest, provide light stimulation for two minutes before pulling the needle out. If the resonance is not felt in the chest, change the direction of the needle further downward. At this moment, the resonance felt inside the chest would be so pleasant that the patient may possibly exclaim. For the treatment of point K26: Point the needle end innerward, and when it reaches the required depth, pull it out rather slowly.

Effects: When the ailment is mild, it can be alleviated by one treatment or at most by two to three treatments. In the cases of more serious ailment, the first treatment would make the patient comfortable and help him to have a good sleep. Through further treatments, the patient's condition would gradually improve, and he may be cured by ten to fifteen treatments in all.

When the ailment of long duration is cured, it is strongly recommended that the Acupunctural treatment should be continued once in every other week for six months in order to strengthen the weakened body as well as to prevent the recurrence.

If the coughing is complicated, the patient may experience nausea and his heart's activity may thus be weakened. In such a case, the needle insertion at the point, CV14(Figure F.13) should be very effective. This point is located at two inches below the xiphoid process. For the treatment of this point: Insert the needle two fifths of an inch deep and provide some stimulation for one minute before pulling it out.

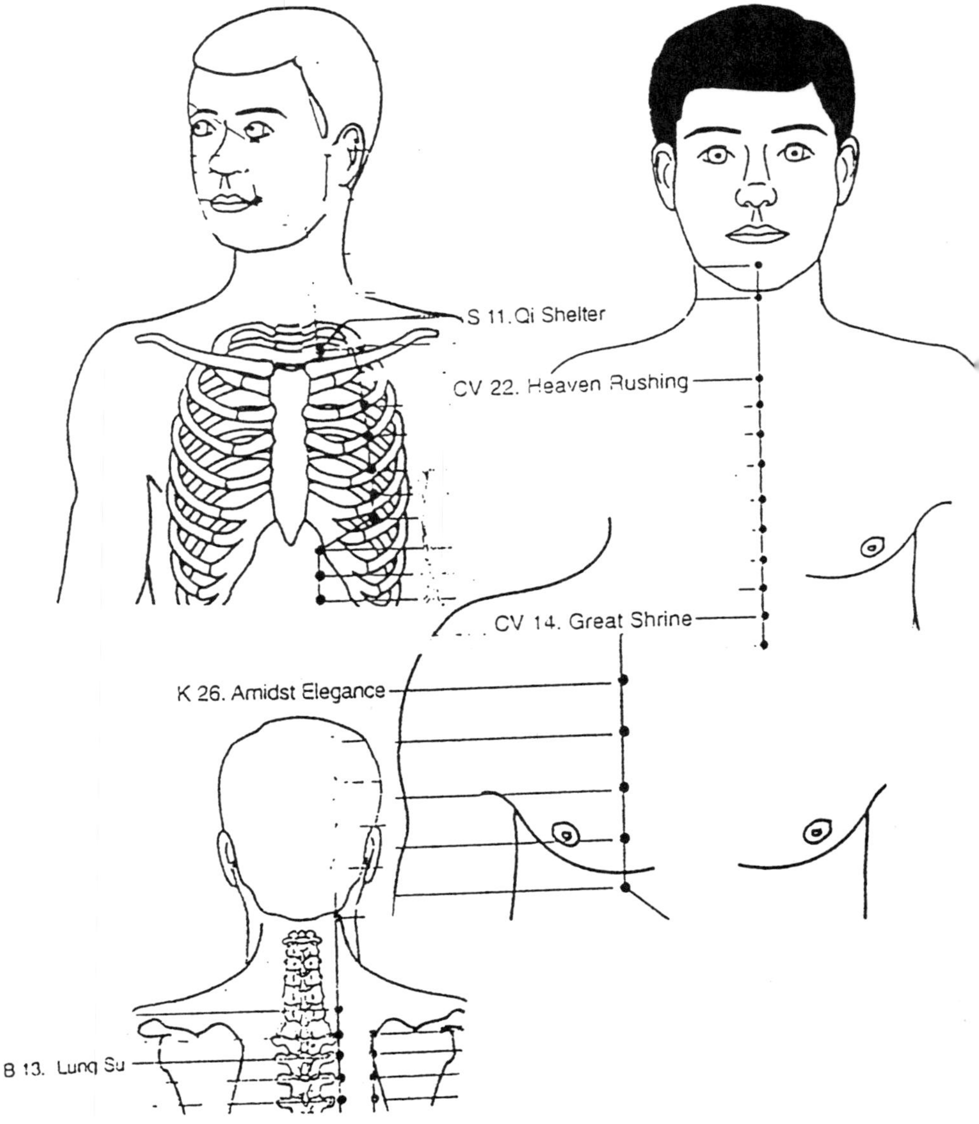
S 11. Qi Shelter
CV 22. Heaven Rushing
CV 14. Great Shrine
K 26. Amidst Elegance
B 13. Lung Su

FIGURE-F13

CHAPTER IV

AILMENT IN BACK SHOULDER

CHAPTER IV
AILMENT IN BACK SHOULDER

1. NEURALGIA IN THE NECK

Neuralgia shows the following symptoms: If one gets up in the morning and suddenly feels pain from the neck to the shoulder;if one finds it very painful and hard to move about his neck or to bend and stretch his neck; and if he lies flat, it is difficult to move his body sideways.
The pain usually occurs to the outer side of the third and fourth cervical vertebrae, or to the outer side of the sixth cervical vertebrae, but sometimes it may come at both of these areas simultaneously.
In the case of the pain around the third and fourth cervical vertebrae, one can easily identify the location of the pain, since when the patient turns his head towards the pained area, he would feel more acute pain or even dizziness. The patient feels pain at the back of the shoulder, when he attempts to move his head up and down or to turn it sideways. In this case, the patient's shoulder pain is associated with the sixth cervical vertebrae. From such observation as described in the above, one will locate exactly where the patient's pain point is. The pain point is, therefore, the Acupuncture point for treatment.

The following two points require Acupunctural treatment:AC1 and AC2, as shown in Figure F.14.

a. AC1:This is the point alongside the third and fourth cervical vertebrae and one and a half inch below the point GB.20.<u>Wind Pond</u> -- one of the commonly applied points.

b. AC2 This is the point located next to the sixth cervical vertebrae. This point can be identified by pressing with fingers. Press the point with fingers and have the patient move his head up and down;if the patient no longer feels the pain, the point is correctly identified.

Depth of Insertion: One half to three fifths of an inch for both points, CV1. and CV2.

Treatment: The patient should be in an upright sitting position. For the treatment of the point CV1.point the needle end inward, and when the needle reaches the proper depth and the resonance is felt at the joint of the occipital bones, provide some stimulation for two or three minutes before extracting the needle. The resonance induced herewith would give the patient a sensational feeling of pleasure. Caution:too strong a resonance may often cause dizziness.
As for the treatment of the point CV2, point the needle downward, and when the needle reaches the prescribed depth and the accompanying resonance is felt around the upper part of the shoulder down to the upper part of the back, provide some stimulation for two or three minutes before extracting the needle.

Effects: In most cases, one treatment should produce a good effect; two treatment s are seldom required.

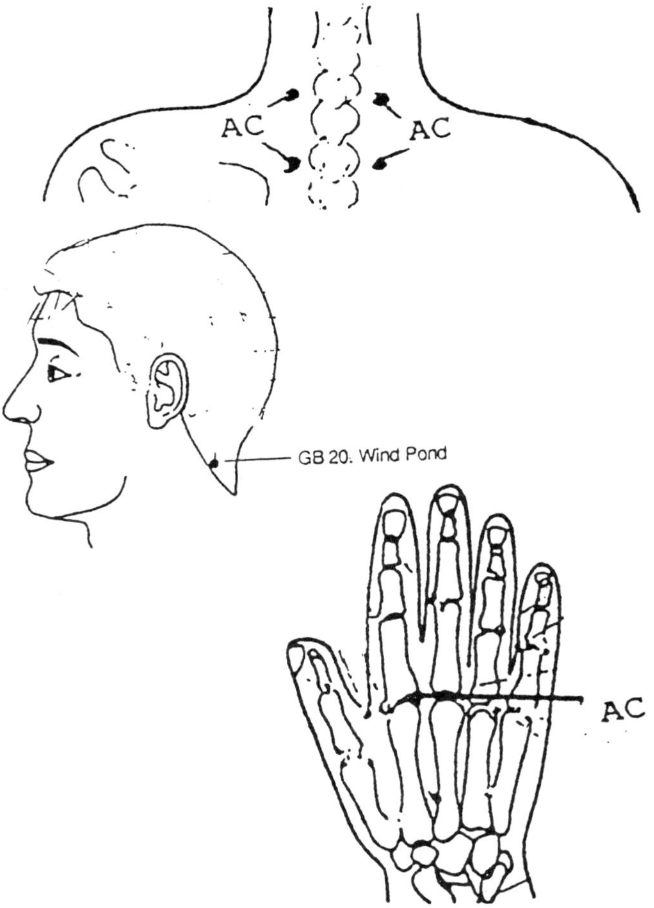

FIGURE- F14

2. PAINS IN THE SHOULDER

Depending upon the areas where the pain and stiffening occur, four categories can be listed.

a. Shoulder pain:The patient always feels pressure and heaviness around the shoulders especially when he attempts to raise his arms.

b. The pain is felt around the upper part of the chest, on either side or on both sides. Right alongside the first and third thoracic vertebrae, there appear some swellings. When the patient attempts to ben his head forward or to turn it to look for the aching part, he would feel a sharp pain and tension in his back.

c. The pain is felt at the middle of the inner edge of the scapula, which corresponds to the middle of the trapezius muscle on each side. If the patient pulls the two scapulas together toward the backbone or if he takes deep breathings, he would feel something uneasy in that area.

d. The pain is felt around the outer edge of the scapula on each side.

Acupunctural points: For the treatment of all four categories of the shoulder pain, as described in the above, the needle insertion should be made on the point which is between the seventh cervical vertebra and the first thoracic vertebra -- just a bit off from the center on each side.

For the treatment of the category (a), the point SI.13.<u>Crooked Wall</u> in Figure F.15 should be utilized. This point is locted at the upper corner of the scapula.

For the treatment of the category (b), the point B12.<u>Wind Gate</u> should be employed. It is found under the second thoracic vertebra, half and inch off to the side.

For the treatment of the category(c), the point B36.<u>Supplement Division</u> and B37.<u>Soul Shelter</u> should be used. This racic vertebra, three inches off toward the outer side, while the point B37. is located half an inch below the point B36,as shown in Figure F.15.

<u>Depth of Insertion</u>: For the point SI.13,the depth should be three fifths or four fifths of an inch. For the point B12, the depth is one half to three fifths of an inch, whereas the depth for the points B36.and B37. is two fifths to one half of an inch.

<u>Treatment</u>:The patient's position should be either sitting straight or lying flat on the stomach. At the point alongside the seventh cervical vertebra, the insertion is made to the prescribed depth while pointing the needle end inward and backward and the resonance is felt firm when the needle reaches the infected area. Provide moderate stimulation for one or two minutes before extracting the needle.
At the points SI.13,BG12,B36, and B37, the resonance would easily reach the infected areas in the back, whereby a pleasant feeling is to be felt by the patient. In treating the point SI.13, point the needle backward so that it hardly touches the front part of the scapula. When the needle gets into the prescribed depth and its resonance reaches the scapula or the armpit, provide light

stimulation in order to provide continuous resonance before extracting the needle.
In treating the point B12, point the needle end inward while pressing the needle into the proper depth. This will generate resonance inside the chest or the neck muscles. Maintain the resonance for two or three minutes by some tapping stimulation before pulling out the needle.
In treating the point B36. or B37,point the needle end forward while inserting the needle with tappings. When the needle reaches the prescribed depth and its resonance is felt firm around the infected areas under the scapula inside the chest, provide some light stimulation for two or three minutes before extracting the needle. Having extracted the needle, the Acupuncturist should press the point with his thumb by gradually increasing pressure; this is a more effective way to alleviate the pain.

Effects:The chronic ailment of sic month to one year duration may be cured by one to three treatments of this kind. Those ailments with longer duration require additional treatments.

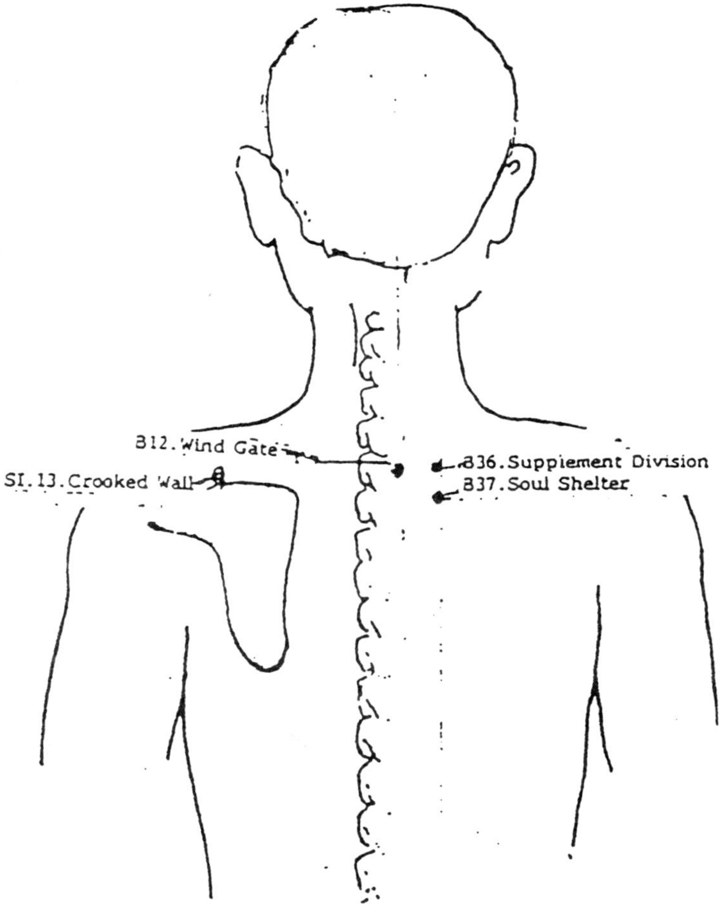
B12. Wind Gate
SI. 13. Crooked Wall
B36. Supplement Division
B37. Soul Shelter

FIGURE - F15

CHAPTER V

AILMENT IN THE HEAD

CHAPTER V
AILMENT IN THE HEAD

1. MEGRIM

Fits of pain ranging from any part of the head up to the top of the head. The attacks occasionally occur on both sides of the head at the same time or alternately on either side.

The Acupunctural points are as follows: See Figure F.16.

a. Point GB.11.Extreme Yin.

Location: Behind the ear on each side at the edge of the bone, termed mastoid process, where an angle or corner is formed at the hair line.

b. Point S8.Head Tied.

Location: This point is located above the forehead on each side. When the teeth are clenched, protrusions are created on the forehead at each side forming the points.

c. points GV.20Hundered Meeting, B10 Heavenly Pillar,GB20.Wind Pond,GB.12 Final Bone,GV.13Kiln Path,B15Heart Su, CV.12Middle Channel,LI.11Crooked Pond, as shown in Figure F.16.

Depth of Insertion: For the point GB11, the depth should be one quarter of an inch. For the point S8,the depth should be one fifth of an inch -- up to the bone.

Treatment: The patient is to be asked to lie o

his side. In treating the point GB.11,aim the needle point out and upward. Insert the needle with slight stimulation. When the needle reaches the proper depth and its resonance is felt at the infected area, leave the needle at the inserted depth for ten minutes. During this time, apply light stimulation for thirty seconds at every two minutes before extracting the needle. The resonance felt at the infected area gives the patient a pleasant sensation. When the resonance is not produced, repeat the above procedure by pointing the needle point up and outward--barely touching the edge of the mastoid bone. This would produce resonance in the infected area of the head. For the treatment of the point S8:When the needle reaches the required depth, apply some stimulation for thirty seconds before pulling it out.

Effects: Acute ailment of this kind is cured by one treatment. The more chronic ones would required three or four treatments--one treatment every other day.

Note: For the treatment of headaches, it is required that the resonance should reach the aching infected area. When the ailment is serious, the patient would feel pain in the eyes and shed tears. IN such a case, the Acupunctural treatment at the point GB.11 would produce resonance in the eyes, which provides the patient with a pleasant sensation and alleviate the pain by preventing the spread of pain to the eyes.

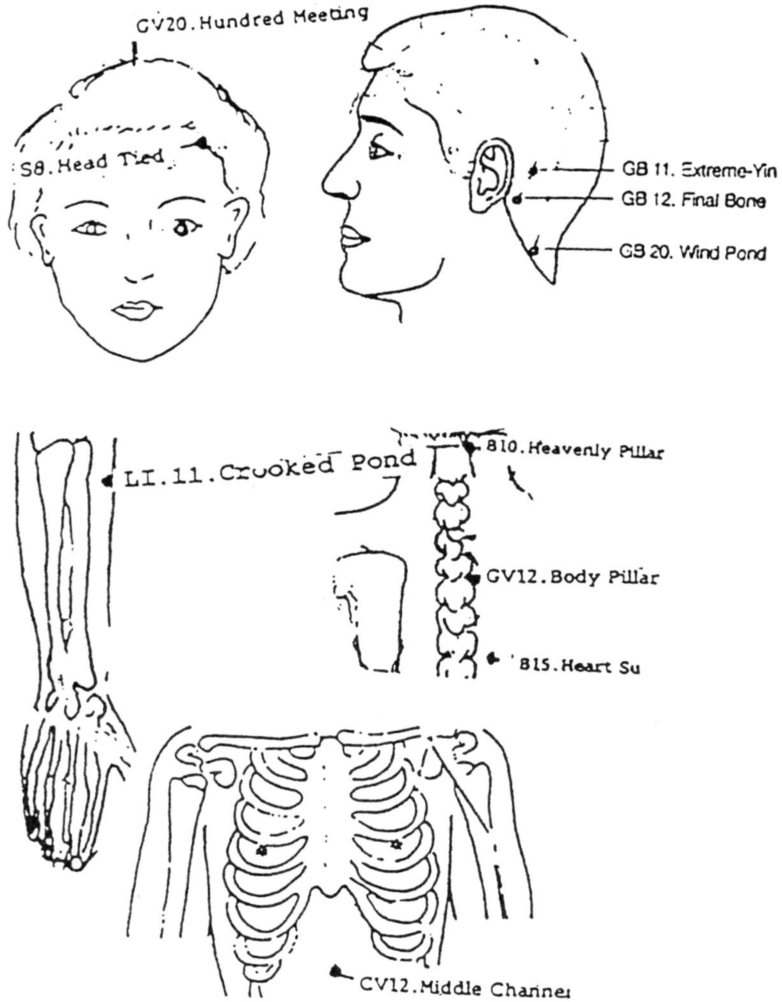
GV20. Hundred Meeting
S8. Head Tied
GB 11. Extreme-Yin
GB 12. Final Bone
GB 20. Wind Pond
LI. 11. Crooked Pond
B10. Heavenly Pillar
GV12. Body Pillar
B15. Heart Su
CV12. Middle Channel

FIGURE- F16

2. OCCIPUT NEURALGIA

Pain spreading from occipital bone over the head on either side or on both side.

The following are the Acupunctural points to be treated, as shown in Figure F.17.

a. Point GB.20Wind Pond:

Location: Under the occipital bone between the two muscles, trapezius and sternocleidomastoid, on each side.

b. Point GB.19Brain Hollow:

Location: About one inch above the point GB.20 on each side.

c. Points GB.11Extreme Yin,B10Heavenly Pillar,upper B10 are also highly recommended.

Depth of Insertion: Point GB.20--one third to four fifths of an inch. Point GB.19--one fifth to a slightly more than one fifth of an inch, reaching up to the bone.

Treatment: The patient should be in a sitting posture. Have the patient sit on the chair with his hands folded on the table and with his forehead resting on his hands. Insert the needle into the skin while aiming its point upward. When the needle gets into the proper depth and its resonance reaches the top of his head, keep the needle in that position for five minutes while providing stimulation tot the needle for twenty seconds every minute. The resonance felt at the top of the head would produce a pleasant sensation.
In treating the point GB.19, insert the needle

down to the bone, and then provide rapid stimulation for one minute before extracting the needle.

Effects: Headache would disappear immediately after the treatment. Acute headaches are cured by a single treatment, whereas the chronic ones are cured by two or three treatments, given every day consecutively, or by five to six treatments, given every other day.

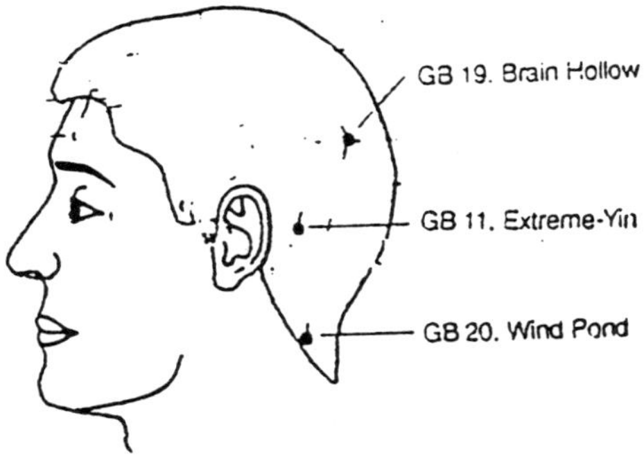
GB 19. Brain Hollow
GB 11. Extreme-Yin
GB 20. Wind Pond

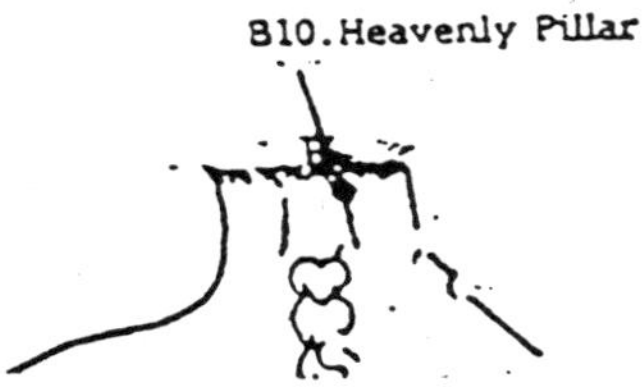
B10. Heavenly Pillar

FIGURE- F17

3. TOOTHACHE

For the treatment of toothache with swollen bums, the following Acupunctural points should be utilized, as shown in Figure F.18.

a. Point SI.17Heavenly Appearance: This point is used for both upper and lower teeth.

Location: Below the ear on each side of the head alongside the mandible bone there is a muscle. Under the muscle is the point for Acupuncture.

b. At the root of the aching tooth.

Depth of Insertion: One half to three fifths of an inch.

Treatment: Have the patient lie on his side with the infected side up. At the point SE.17, insert the needle at a 30°(degree) angle. When it reaches the proper depth, apple some stimulation for about two minutes and wait until the pain gradually subsides before extracting the needle.

c. For the treatment of the lower set of teeth, insert the needle into the root of the aching tooth by pointing the needle toward the interior of the tooth but not touching the tooth itself. When the needle reaches approximately half an inch in depth, it would arouse a feeling of sensation for two or three minutes; then, keep the needle inserted for a few minutes and apply some more stimulation before pulling the needle out. It is mandatory in this treatment that the resonance must reach the aching spot so as to provide the patient with a sense of comfort.

d. When any of the upper teeth aches, the needle insertion should be aimed at the root of the aching tooth. When the needle's end reaches the root of the tooth, apply some light stimulation and, after witnessing that the pain disappears, extract the needle. This treatment takes about two or three minutes.

Effects: Usually one treatment should suffice, but occasionally it requires one additional treatment.

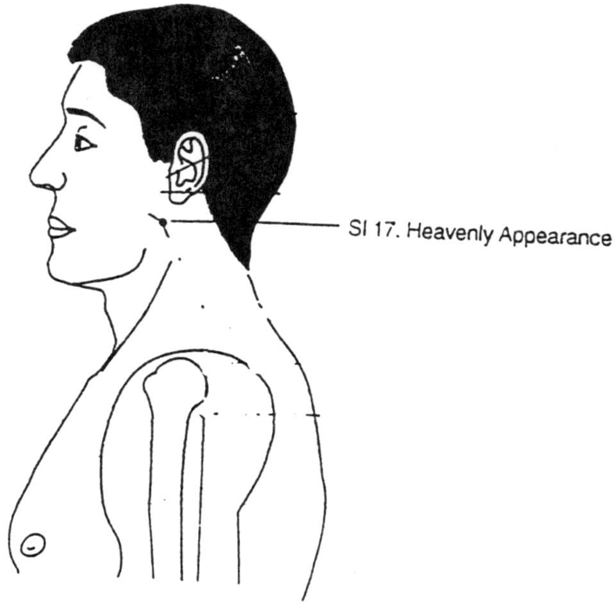

FIGURE- F18

4. TRIGEMINAL NEURALGIA

This ailment causes the pain around the forehead, above and below the eyes, or around the chin.

The following are the Acupunctural points to be treated, as shown in Figure F.19.

a. Point GB.11Extreme Yin

B. Point GB.14Yang White

c. Point GV.22Upper Star and B2Drilling Bamboo are also in common usage.

Location: Right above the center of each eyebrow, where there is a little hollow in the bone on each side of the forehead.

Depth of Insertion: Between on tenth and two tenths of an inch.

Treatment: For the treatment of the point 14, ask the patient to lie flat on his back and provide a pillow to support his neck. Insert the needle until it slightly touches the bone. Provide some light stimulation to the needle for one or two minutes before pulling it out. When the needle point slightly touches the bone, the patient would feel a pleasant sensation. It is recommended that any stronger stimulation should be avoided.

Effects: The headache disappears right after the treatment. Acute ailment can be cured by one treatment.

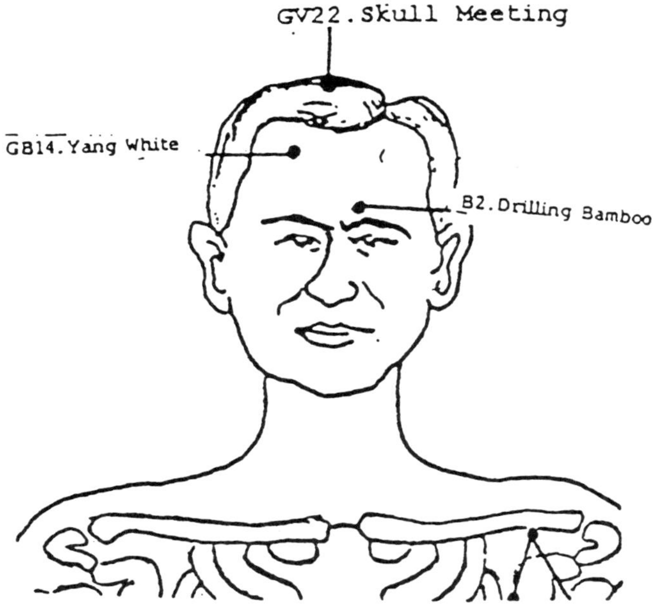
GV22. Skull Meeting
GB14. Yang White
B2. Drilling Bamboo

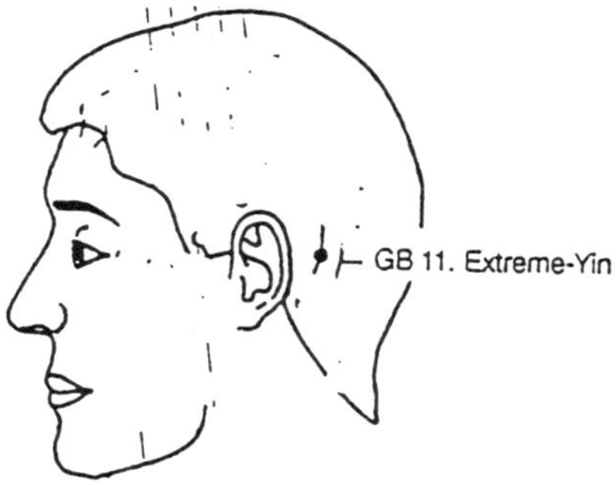
GB 11. Extreme-Yin

FIGURE- F19

5. THE EYE AILMENTS

Declining eyesight, tears, pain in the eyes, glaucoma, near-sightedness, conjunctivitis,etc. are the general symptoms under this category.

The following Acupunctural points should be utilized, as illustrated in Figure F.20.

a. Point GB.11Extreme Yin(See MEGRIM Section)

b. Point GB.Eye Bone: Located just above the corner of the eye.

c. Point B2Drilling Bamboo:One can feel a little hollow spot in the bone just above the edge of the eyebrow.

c. Points LI.11Crooked Pond,B12Wind Gate, GV.13Kiln Path.

Depth of Insertion: For the point GB1,one half or three fifths of an inch in depth. For the point B2, one and one tenth of an inch.

Treatment: Have the patient lie flat on his back. For treating the point GB.11, the needle point should be aimed outward and upward while pressing the needle with moderate stimulation. At the prescribed depth, when the resonance is felt in the eyes, apply steady pressure. If the first insertion fails to yield resonance in the eye corners, repeat the above procedures two or three times or change the direction of the needle point in order to produce the resonance in the eye.
For treating the point GB.1, the needle end should be aimed downward and forward. When the needle reaches a proper depth, keep the inserted needle there for two or three

minutes. During this time, provide a few light stimulation before extracting the needle. For the treatment of the point B2, the needle end should be aimed upward while inserting it with a very light stimulation. When the needle end barely touches the bone, provide a few tapping stimulation before pulling the needle out.

<u>Effects</u>: The weakening of eyesight, tears, pain in the eye corners, conjunctivitis can be cured by two or three separate treatments. Other kinds of ailments may be cured by ten separate treatments or more.

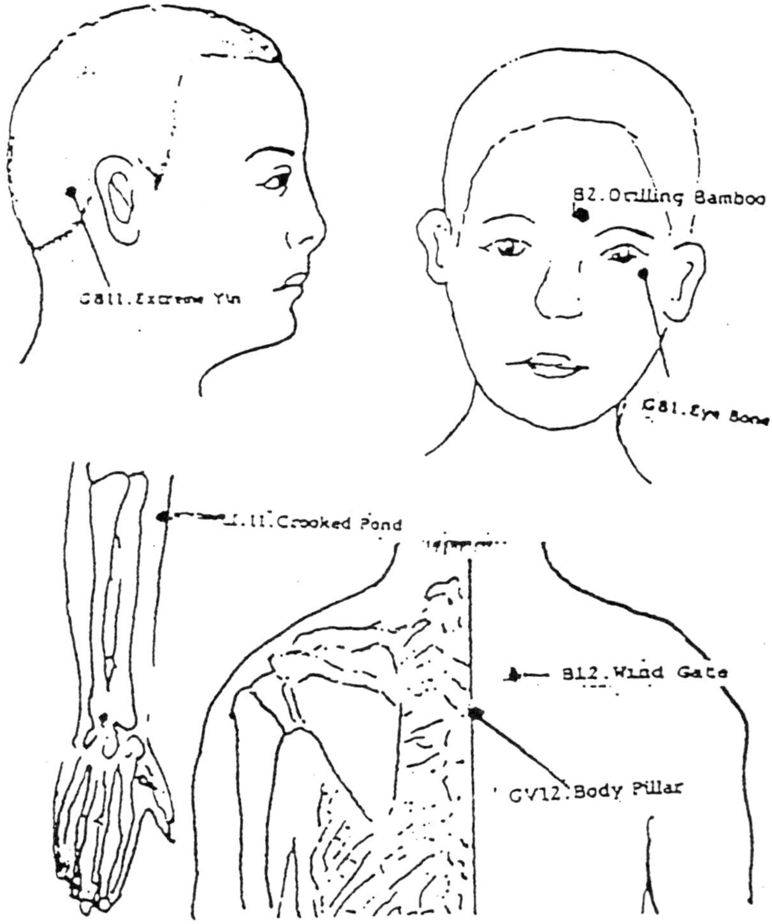
B2. Drilling Bamboo
Extreme Yin
Eye Bone
11. Crooked Pond
B12. Wind Gate
GV12. Body Pillar

FIGURE-F20

6. THE EAR AILMENTS

Acute inflammation of the mid ear, otosclerosis(buzzing in the ear), paints in the ear, etc., are the general ailments of the ear.

Acupunctural points to be used are as follows:(See Figure F.21).

a. Point SI.17Heavenly Appearance.

Location: Behind the ear right below the mastoid process, where the muscle platysma originates.

b. Point T17Wind Screen.

Location: At the hollow point between the ear and the mastoid process.

c. Point T18Feeding Meriding.

Location: Half an inch above the point T17 behind the ear on the mastoid process bone. If this point is pressed, a pressing bivration in the ear is felt. This point is particularly effective for treating the earache.

d. Points K6Shining Sea and H3Lesser Sea are also commonly utilized.

Depth of Insertion: For the point SI.17: in the cases of acute inflammation of the mid ear and earaches, one third to one half of an inch is preferable, while for other kinds of ear ailments four fifths to one full inch is recommended.
For the point T17: In the cases of acute

inflammation of the mid ear, one fifth to one third of an inch, whereas for other kinds of ear ailments, one third to one half of an inch.
For the point T18: One tenth to one seventh of an inch--barely up to the bone.

Treatment: Have the patient lie on his side with the infected ear upside. For the treatment of the point SI17, aim the needle point forward and upward and, when the needle reaches the proper depth and its resonance is felt inside of the ear, stop further insertion. Give some light stimulation before extracting the needle. Repeat the above treatment for two or three minutes. It is recommended that needle stimulation should be as mild as possible for acute inflammation of the mid ear and earaches, whereas a bit stronger stimulation should be applied for treating other kinds of ear ailment.
For the treatment of the point T17, when the needle reaches a certain depth, provide continuous light stimulation for two minutes before pulling the needle out. It must be strongly emphasized that stimulation should not be too strong.
For the treatment of the point T18: When the needle point slightly touches the bone, provide a light stimulation for one or two minutes before extracting the needle. This Acupunctural point is very effective for treating ear ailments.

Effects: In the cases of acute inflammation and earaches, the aching feeling ceases immediately after the treatment, but the complete alleviation of ear inflammation requires three or four successive treatments. One treatment should be given every day. In the case of chronic inflammation, the fluid stops after one to three separate treatments.

If ailments such as hearing defects, buzzing the ears, ear fluid had lasted for more than a year before the treatment, ten or more separate treatments are necessary t alleviate them.

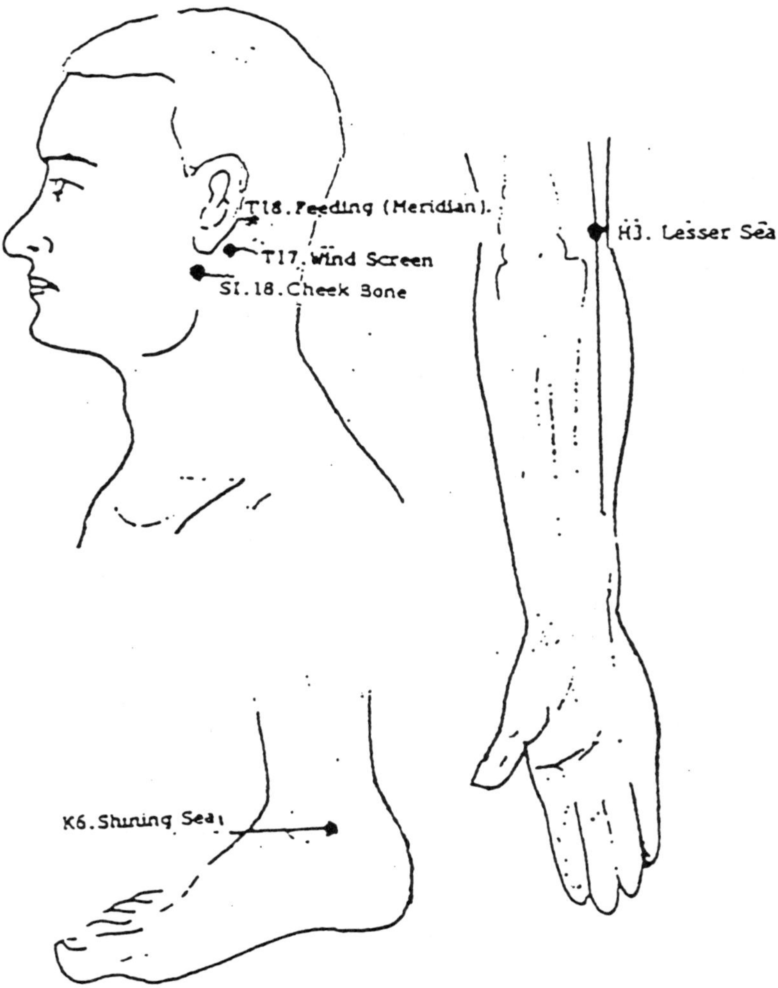

FIGURE- F21

7. THE NOSE AILMENTS

Nose catarrh, ozena, ear blockade, swollen and inflamed mucous membranes,etc., are the common ailments of the nose.

The following are the Acupunctural points for treatment, as shown in Figure F.22.

Points GB.20Wind Pond,B2Drilling Bamboo,and LI.20Welcome Fragrance.

Location: At the base of the nose, at the side of the nose, and right above the back neck, as seen in Figure F.22.

Depth of Insertion:One third or one half of an inch.

Treatment: Have the patient lie flat on his back with a pillow supporting his neck. Insert the needle with its point aiming a bit inward. When the needle reaches one third of an inch in depth, provide tapping stimulation for thirty seconds, and then push the needle one tenth of an inch deeper by piercing through any obstacle while providing some more stimulation. When the needle point come in contact with the bone, stop any further insertion there and give stimulation for one more minute before pulling the needle out.

Effects: If the ailment is not a chromic one, two or three separate treatments should suffice to stop the snivelling, to open the blocked nasal openings, and to recover the normal state in the head. If the ailment is of many years' duration, about ten separate treatments are required.

Note: This point is very sensitive for the treatment of ozena. The resonance would reach into the nose, thereby providing a good feeling. The longer the duration of the ailments, the better the patient would feel, and the chocking feeling in the nose would disappear in seconds after the treatment.

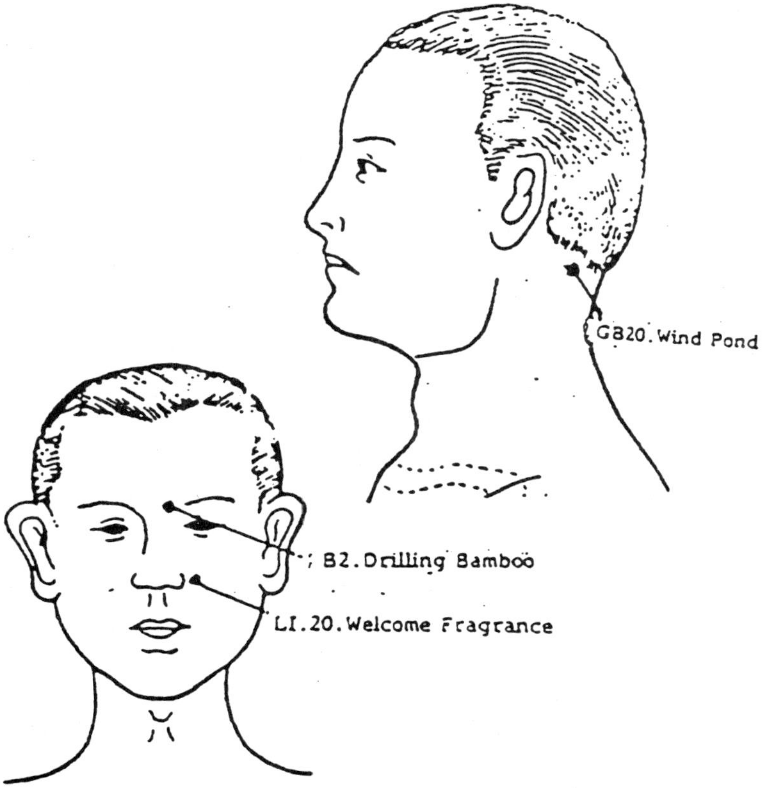

FIGURE- F22

8. INSOMNIA

The main symptom is that the patient can hardly sleep. Even if he does sleep, he can be easily awakened by slight noises or disturbance in the dreams--mostly nightmares.

The following are the Acupunctural points for treatment, as shown in Figure F.23.

a. Point B10Heavenly Pillar.

Location: The point B10 is located under the occipital bone between the first and the second cervical vertebrae on each side of the back neck.

b. Point B2Drilling Bamboo,B17 Diaphragm Su,H7Spirit Door,etc.

Depth of Insertion: For serious cases, which are very sensitive, a shallow insertion is required--one third of an inch in depth. When the case is not so serious and less sensitive, one half or three fifths of an inch is recommended.

Treatment: It is more convenient for the treatment to have the patient in a lying flat rather than in a sitting position. Aim the needle straight down and insert it into the skin up to the prescribed depth. Then, provide rapid but mild stimulation for two minutes. It is not necessary to produce resonance in other area through any stronger stimulation. through slow stimulation the patient would receive a pleasant feeling.

Effects: The patient tends to fall asleep during the treatment. The ailments of short duration can be cured by one treatment. this means that the patient can sleep normally without nightmares. Such sysmbtoms as dizziness, insomnia, and neurasthenia have their sensitive spots at this point. When the ailments are serious the related sensitive spots develop in a line above the neck as much as one inch in length. The patient would feel tension at the back on the neck and thus feel dizzy.

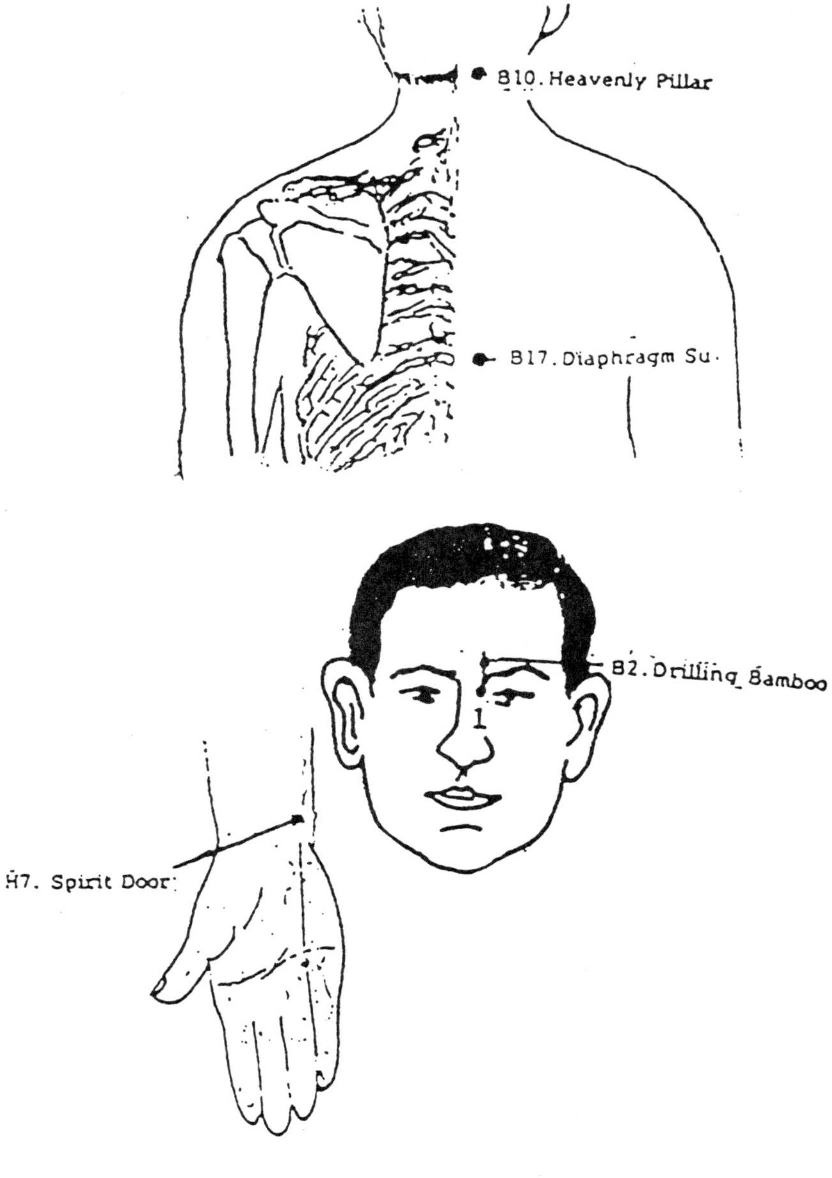
B10. Heavenly Pillar
B17. Diaphragm Su.
B2. Drilling Bamboo
H7. Spirit Door

FIGURE- F23

CHAPTER VI

AILMENTS OF THE ABDOMEN

CHAPTER VI
AILMENTS OF THE ABDOMEN

1. <u>THE BLADDER CATARRH</u>

This ailment causes the following symptoms. The patient feels pain in the bladder head whenever he urinates. After urination, the patient may still feel uncomfortable;he may feel an urge to urinate more.

The following are the Acupunctural points, as illustrated in Figure F.24.

a. Point CV.3<u>Middle Extreme</u>.

<u>Location</u>: Two inches above the junction of the pubis bones.

b. Other points:LV.8<u>Crooked Spring</u>,K12<u>Big Brightness</u>,and B33<u>Middle Bone</u>.

<u>Depth of insertion:</u> Four fifths of an inch to one inch in depth.

<u>Treatment</u>: Have the patient lie flat on his back with his arms and legs stretched outward. Insert the needle vertically into the skin and when the resonance is felt from the bottom to the head of the bladder, stop the insertion and provide stimulation. Give stimulation for one minute, and then stop it for thirty seconds;repeat this procedure two or three more times before extracting the needle. Then the resonance is felt in the neck of the bladder, the patient would feel a sensation.

<u>Effects</u>: This ailment is usually cured by two to three separate treatments.

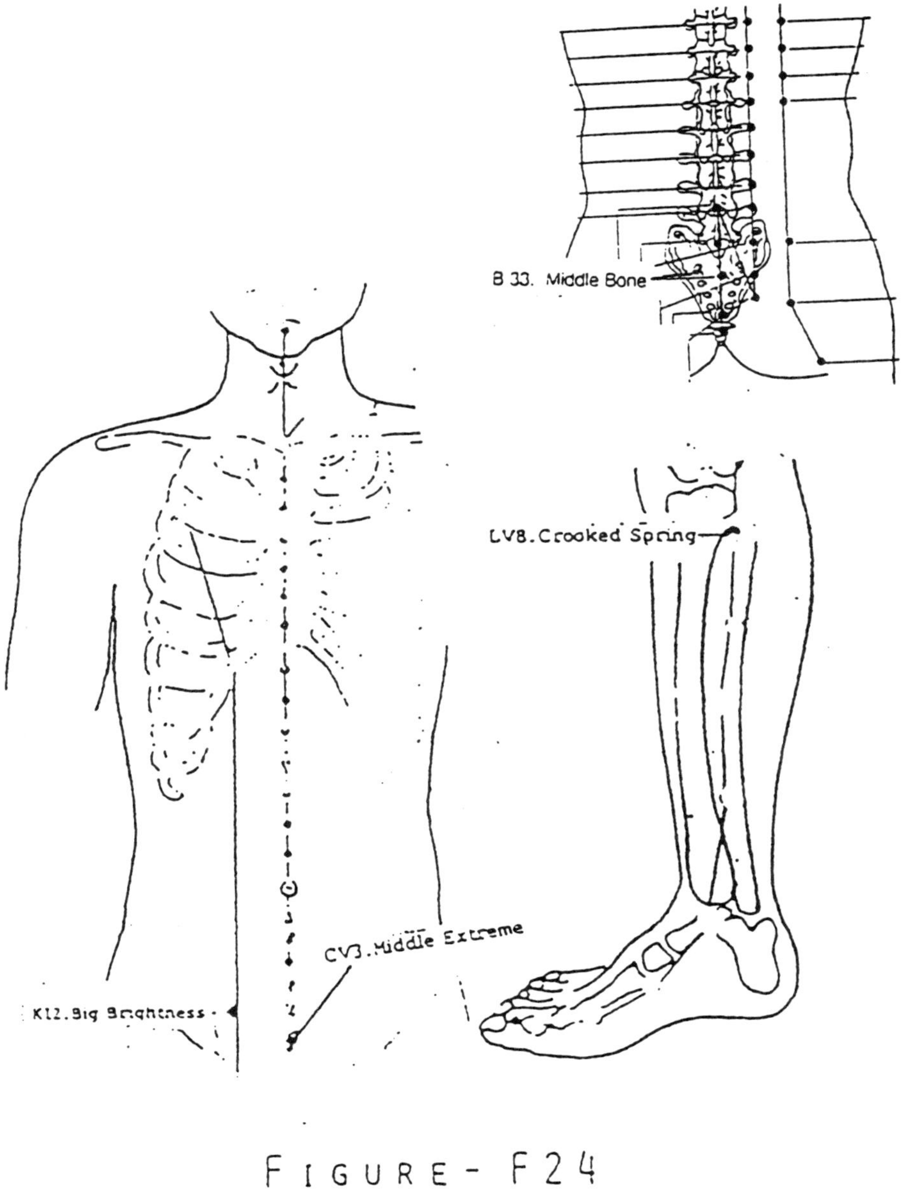
B 33. Middle Bone
LV8. Crooked Spring
CV3. Middle Extreme
K12. Big Brightness

FIGURE- F24

2. BED WETTING

Children, aged four or five, may urinate during the sleep, and are simply unable to control urination.

Acupunctural point for such an ailment is as follows(See Figure F.25):

a. Point CV.3Middle Extreme.

Location and Treatment: See the Section on Bladder Catarrh.

Effects: It is cured by several treatments--one for every other day.

Note: The treatment of the point CV.3 is proved to quite effective for excessive urge to urinate.

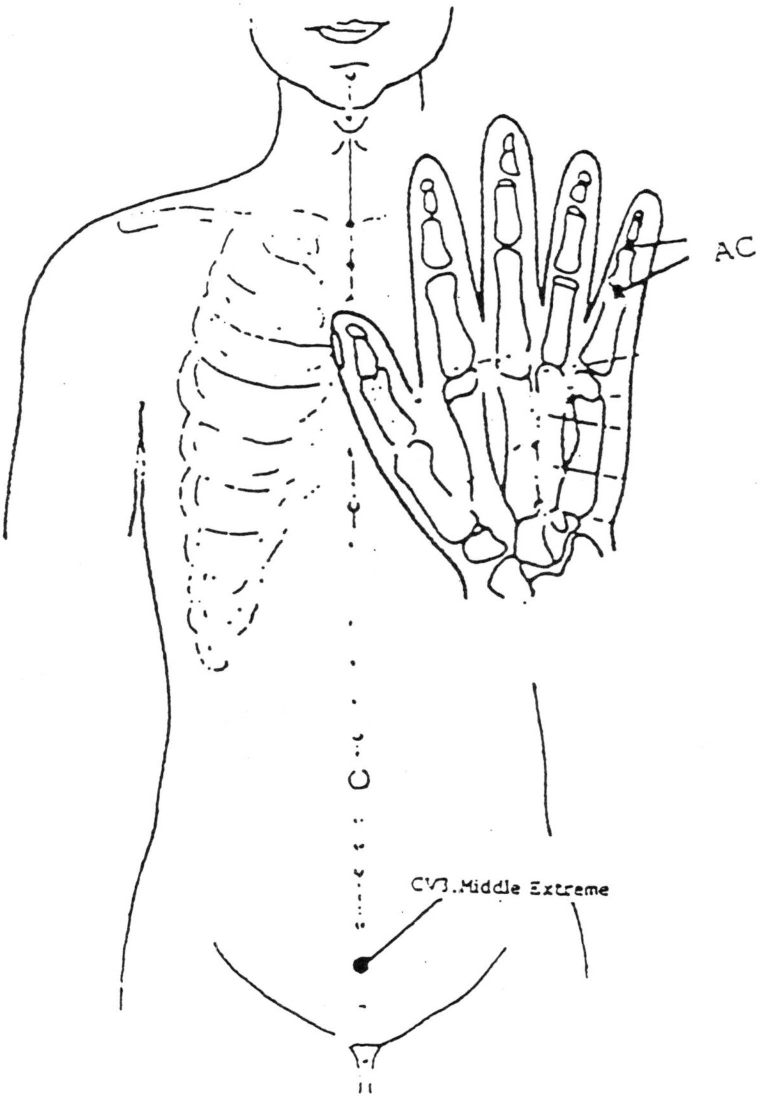

FIGURE- F25

3. NAUSEA

Nausea usually occurs in connection with the ailments of the stomach and intestine or in connection with the disturbance in the nervous system. Nausea may occur due to peritonitis, the diseases of women, or the presence of roundworm. Sever cough can also causes nausea.

For Acupuncture treatment, the following three pints are usually utilized:CV.13Upper Channel on the stomach,T9Four Gutters and T5Outer Gate on the hands.

Treatment: For the treatment of nausea associated with the ailments of the stomach and intestine, the points S19No Admittance,B17 Diaphragm Su,and B45Stomach Granary(See Figure F.26) are used. For the treatment of nausea associated with the disturbed nervous system, the points GV.21Anterior Summit,CV.17Platform Middle,B18Liver Su,and B45Stomach Granary are employed. For the treatment of nausea caused by other ailments, the points CV.12Middle Channel, B20Spleen Su,S9Man Welcome, CV.14 Great Shrine,S36Leg Three Miles,LI.10Arm Three Miles,and B46Vitals Door in Figure F.46 are usually utilized.

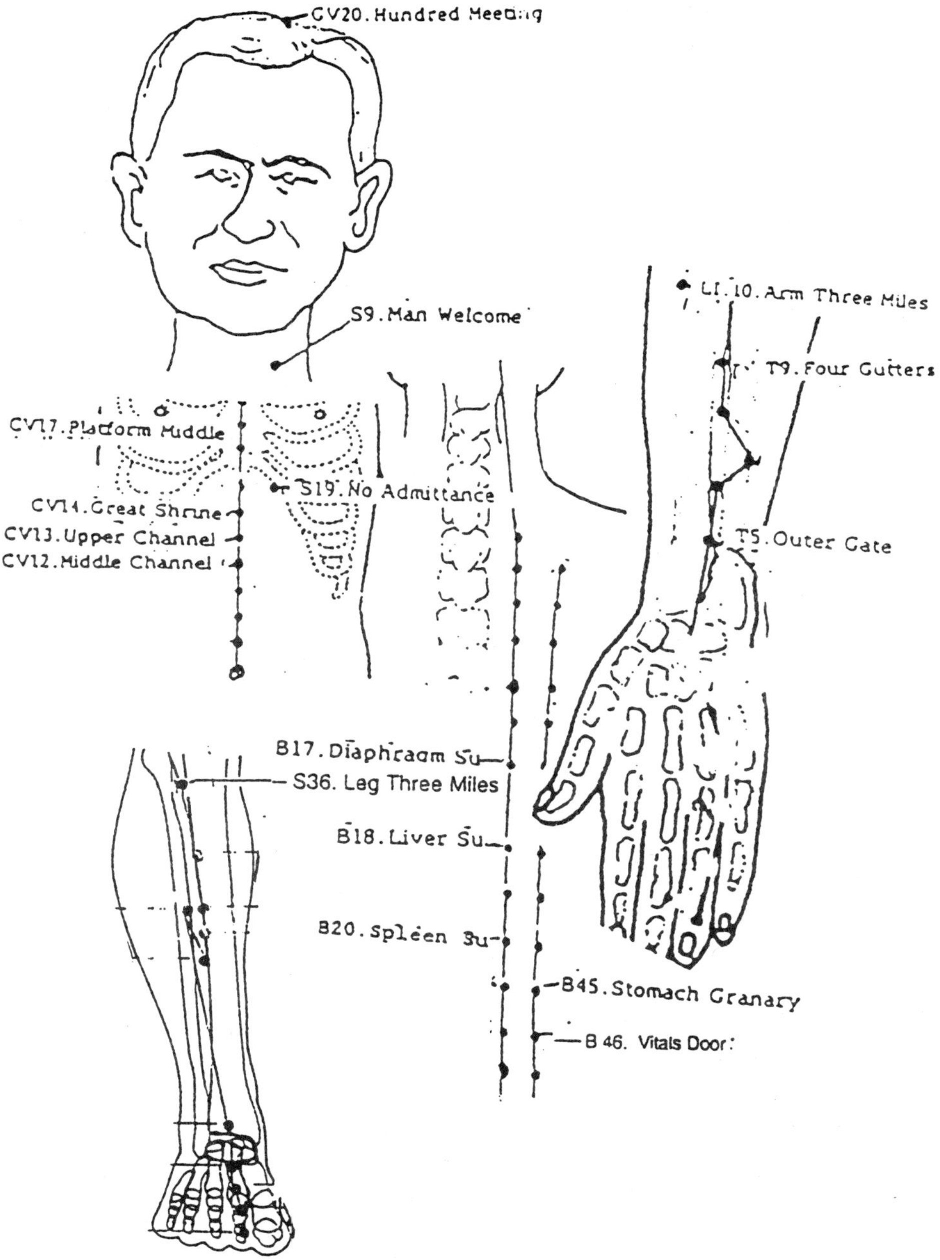
CV20. Hundred Meeting
S9. Man Welcome
CV17. Platform Middle
S19. No Admittance
CV14. Great Shrine
CV13. Upper Channel
CV12. Middle Channel
LI. 10. Arm Three Miles
T9. Four Gutters
T5. Outer Gate
B17. Diaphragm Su
S36. Leg Three Miles
B18. Liver Su
B20. Spleen Su
B45. Stomach Granary
B 46. Vitals Door

FIGURE - F26

4. PAINS IN THE STOMACH

The following treatments are for the general ailments of the stomach, such as stomach ulcers, the falling of the stomach, stomach catarrh, convulsion in the stomach, acid dyspepsia, etc.

These are the Acupunctural points to be treated, as shown in Figure F.27.

a. Point CV.12Middle Channel.

Location: At the mid point between the xiphoid process and the naval.

b. Point CV.16Middle Courtyard.

Location: Half an inch below the xiphoid process(This point is very sensitive in the cases of chronic stomach ailments. Accordingly, this point is used for the diagnosis of stomach ailments).

Depth of Insertion: For the point CV.12, the proper depth of insertion is three fifths to four fifths of an inch. In the cases of stomach ulcers and stomach catarrhs, one third to one half of an inch is recommended. For the point CV.16, one fifth of an inch is recommended.

Treatment: Have the patient lie flat on his back with his hands and legs outstretched. For the treatment of the point CV.12, insert the needle vertically into the skin(pressing down while turning the point upward) and when it reaches the required depth, provide some stimulation for two or three minutes before pulling the needle out. The resonance would be felt inside the chest--providing the patient with a pleasant sensation and producing a churning feeling in the stomach. In the cases of the stomach ulcer and stomach catarrh, give a few additional insertions around the point CV.12;the depth should be three tenths to four fifths of an inch(for a thin person, one fifths to three tenths of an inch) and some stimulation be given.

For the treatment of the point CV.16, insert the needle into the proper depth and provide some stimulation for one or two minutes before extracting the needle. Through this treatment, the patient would feel relieved of a blocking feeling in the chest.Give some mild stimulation to the needle tip for one or two minutes before pulling the needle out.

Effects: Acute stomach pains or those ailments connected with the disturbed nervous system can be cured by one treatment. Other chronic stomach ailments required ten separate treatments--one given in every other day.

Note: for such symptoms as stomach expansion or heartburn, the Acupuncture treatment on the points CV.16 and CV.12 proved to be remarkably effective. For the treatment of the lack of appetite,the insertion at the point CV.12 is effective. We have often seen some patients cured by one single treatment,and these patients had been suffering from lost appetite for several months.

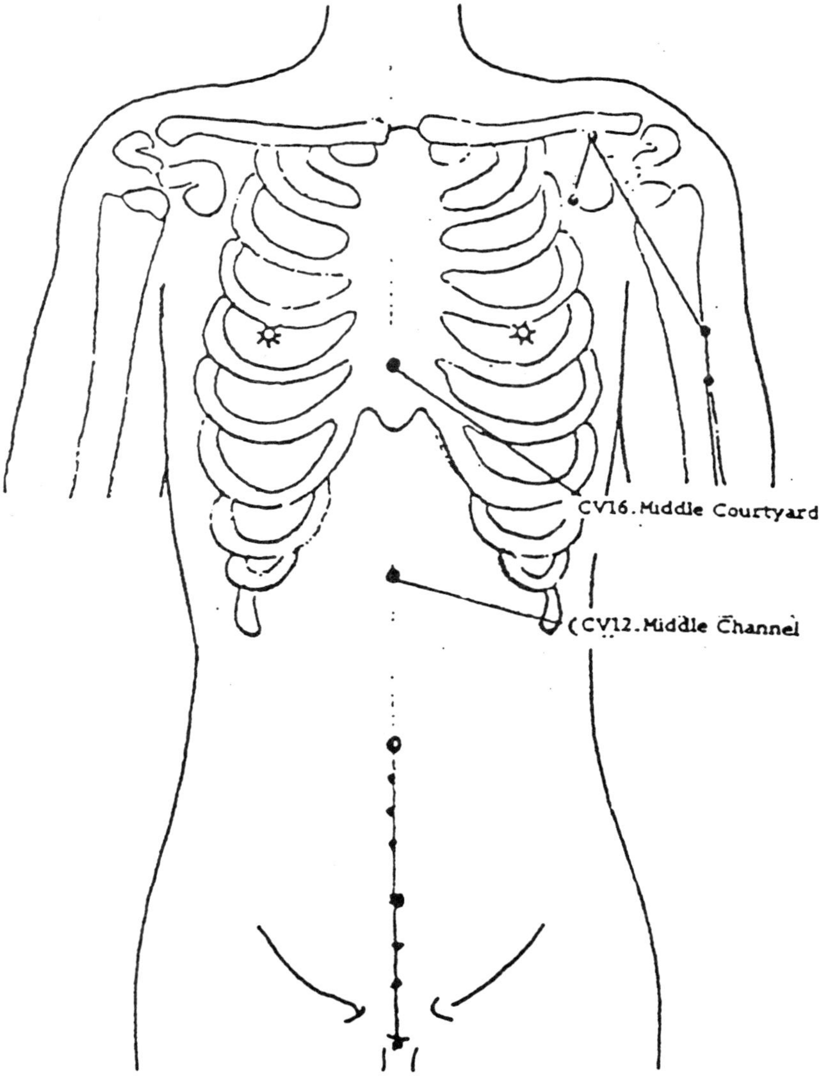

FIGURE-F27

5. CHRONIC LARGE INTESTINE CATARRH

Any patient with this ailment would feel pain in the lower abdomen whenever he tries to evacuate, and he would have bowel movement five or six times a day. Moreover, he would feel pressure in the lower abdomen, which makes him feel like having a bowel movement.

The following Acupunctural points should be employed, as shown in Figure F.28.

a. Point CV.4Gate Origin.

Location: At three inches below the naval.

b. Point B26Gate Origin Su.

Location: One fifth of an inch from the center line under the lumbar vertebra on each side.

c. Points CV.12Middle Channel,S36LegThree Miles, B46Vitals Door,B21Stomach Su, B20Spleen Su ,and S21Beam Door.

Depth of Insertion: For the point CV.4,one inch to one and three tenths of an inch. for the point B26,seven tenths to eight tenths of an inch in depth.

Treatment: For the treatment of the point CV.4 as shown in Figure F.28, the patient position should be lying flat on his back with his hands and legs outstretched. Press the needle reaches the proper depth and its resonance is felt around the anus, stop further insertion and provide some light stimulation for one minute--then pose for thirty seconds. Repeat the above procedure by providing similar stimulation three more times before extracting the needle.

Through the treatments like these, the resonance would reach the anus and thus produce its remarkable effects. If the resonance does not occur in the anus, try to produce the resonance in some other way, as explained below.

Example: Pull the needle out and insert again by changing the spot. Repeat this procedure two or three more times. When the resonance finally reaches the anus, it would yield a very pleasant sensation.

The depth at which the resonance is produced varies according to different individuals, but the resonance commonly occurs at the depth of seven tenths of an inch. For some patients, however, the resonance would not occur until the needle reaches one inch depth.

For the treatment of the point B26Gate Origin Su,have the patient lie on his stomach with his forehead resting on his folded hands. Insert the needle by pointing its end downward inside the skin until it reaches the required depth. Provide moderate stimulation for one or two minutes and then pull the needle out; the resonance would be felt inside the ilium.

Effects: the ailment of this kind can be cured by one to three separate treatments.It rarely requires more than three treatments even for the ailments of long duration.

Note: The Acupunctural treatment of the point CV.4 is surprisingly effective for such symptom as constipation lower abdominal expansion. We had sometimes observed some patients, who having had no bowel movement for a few days, excrete a few hours after the first treatment.

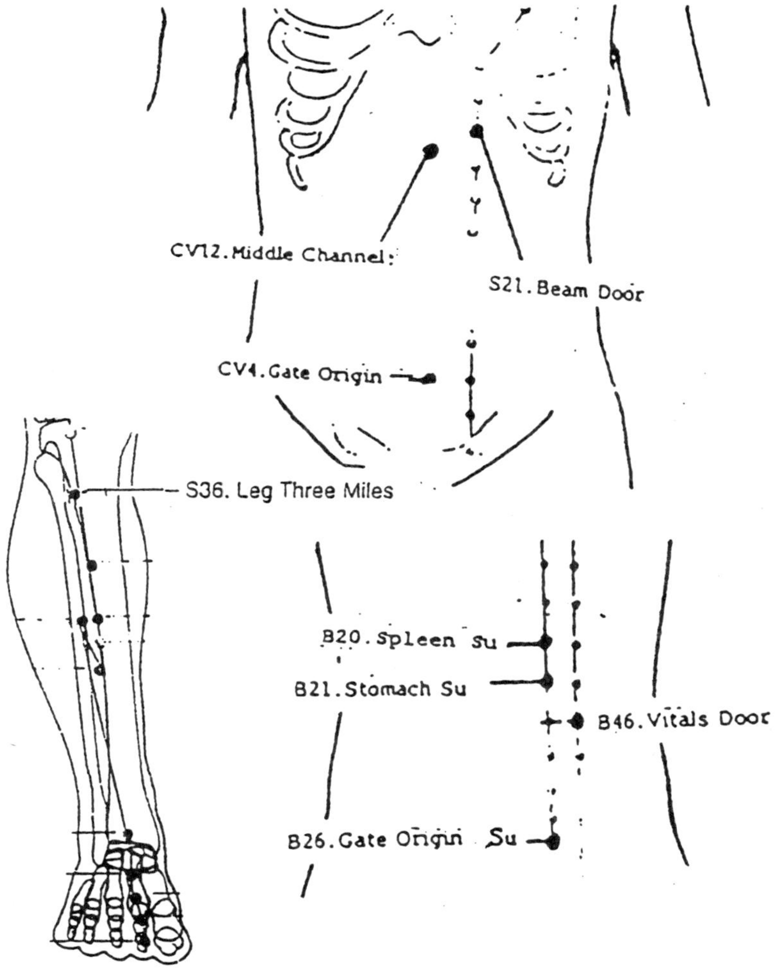

FIGURE- F28

6. PILES

The patient has pain and is bleeding when eliminating, because of the blood congestion in the vein at the anus. Something like a lump (large or small) has developed at the anus, which produces pain when the patient attempts to walk or sit.

The following Acupunctural points are recommended, as shown in Figure F.29.

a. Point CV.4Gate Origin.

Location: See the Section on Large Intestine Catarrh.

b. Point B35Meeting of the Yang.

Location: At the end of the ischium--a little away toward outside on each side.

c. Poins B33Middle Bone, B34Lower Bone, and

B25Large Intestine Su (for relieving constipation).

Depth of Insertion: One half to three fifths of an inch.

Treatment: Have the patient lie on his stomach with his legs wide stretched at a 45 degree angle. For the treatment of the point CV.4, insert the needle rather upward, and when it reaches the prescribed depth, provide light stimulation for one or two minutes before extracting the needle. through the repetition of two or three more treatments at the same Acupunctural point, better results would often appear. The resonance would be felt in the muscle of the anus, and this provide the patient with a pleasant sensation. Having extracted the needle, it would be better to press the insertion points on both sides with your thumbs.

Effects: The pain is usually relieved by one treatment, and the pain is completely gone one or two hours after such a treatment. When the patient has a lump around the anus, a few days are needed for it to dry into a scab, which will then be detached from the skin. During this process, the patient would feel no pain at all.

Note: The treatment of B35 would be very effective for the prolapse of the anus as well.

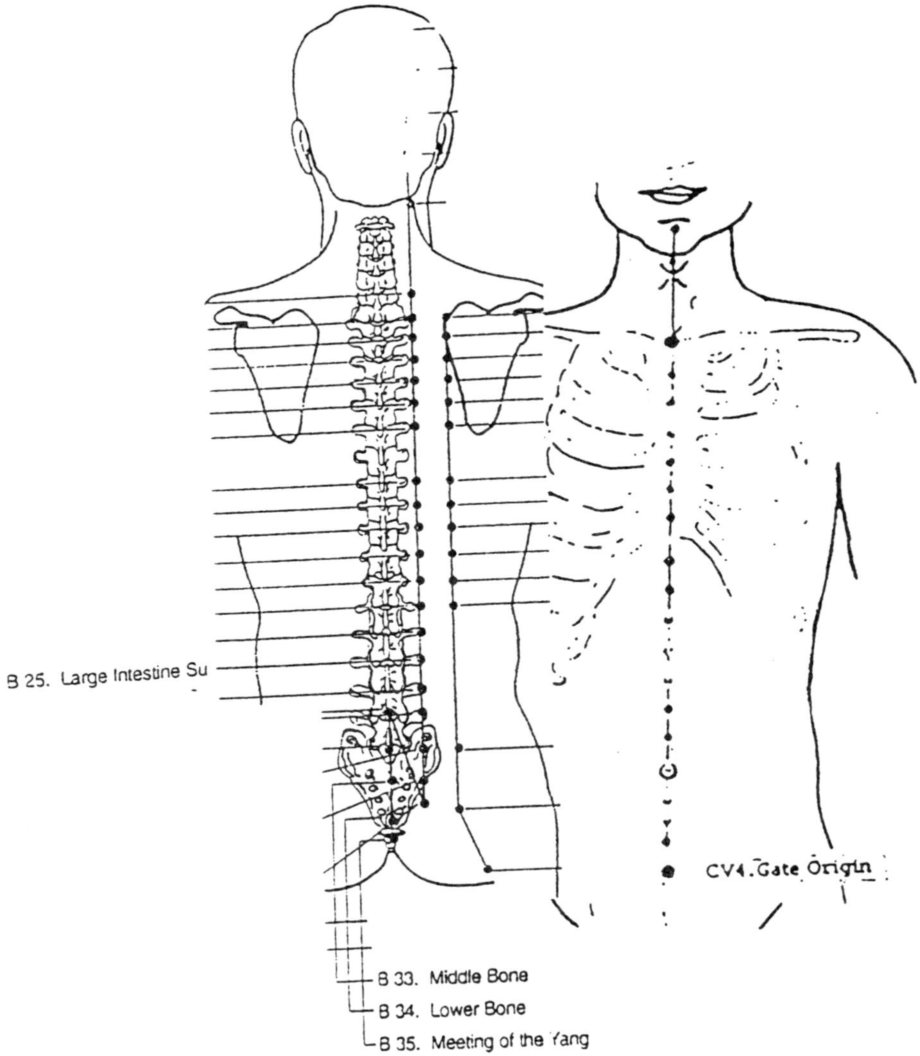
B 25. Large Intestine Su
CV4. Gate Origin
B 33. Middle Bone
B 34. Lower Bone
B 35. Meeting of the Yang

FIGURE- F29

7. ORCHITIS

The symptom involved swollen and painful testicles. When the patient attempts to walk or sit, he would feel severe pain in the testicles, together with pain of contraction in the lower abdomen.

The following Acupunctural pints are recommended, as illustrated in Figure F.30/

a. Point CV.3Middle Extreme.

Location and Treatment: See the Section on Bladder Catarrh.

b. Point S30Rushing Qi.

Location: Two inches off from the center line in the lower abdomen, just below where one can feel the pulse of the femoral artery.

c. Point B26Gate Origin Su.

Location: See the Section on Chronic Large Intestine.

Depth of Insertion: For the point CV.3,Four fifths of an inch to one inch in depth. For the point S, one inch to one and three tenths of an inch. For the point B26, seven tenths to eight tenths of an inch in depth.

Treatment: Have the patient lie flat on his back with his arms and legs outstretched. Insert the needle downward, and when needle reaches the proper depth and its resonance is felt at the testicles, provide light stimulation for thirty seconds and pose for one minute. Repeat this treatment two or three more times, and then pull the needle out.

Effects: Acute orchitis can be cured by three or four separate treatments--one treatment every day. Chronic orchitis with more than one year's duration can be cured by ten separate treatments--providing one treatment in every other day.

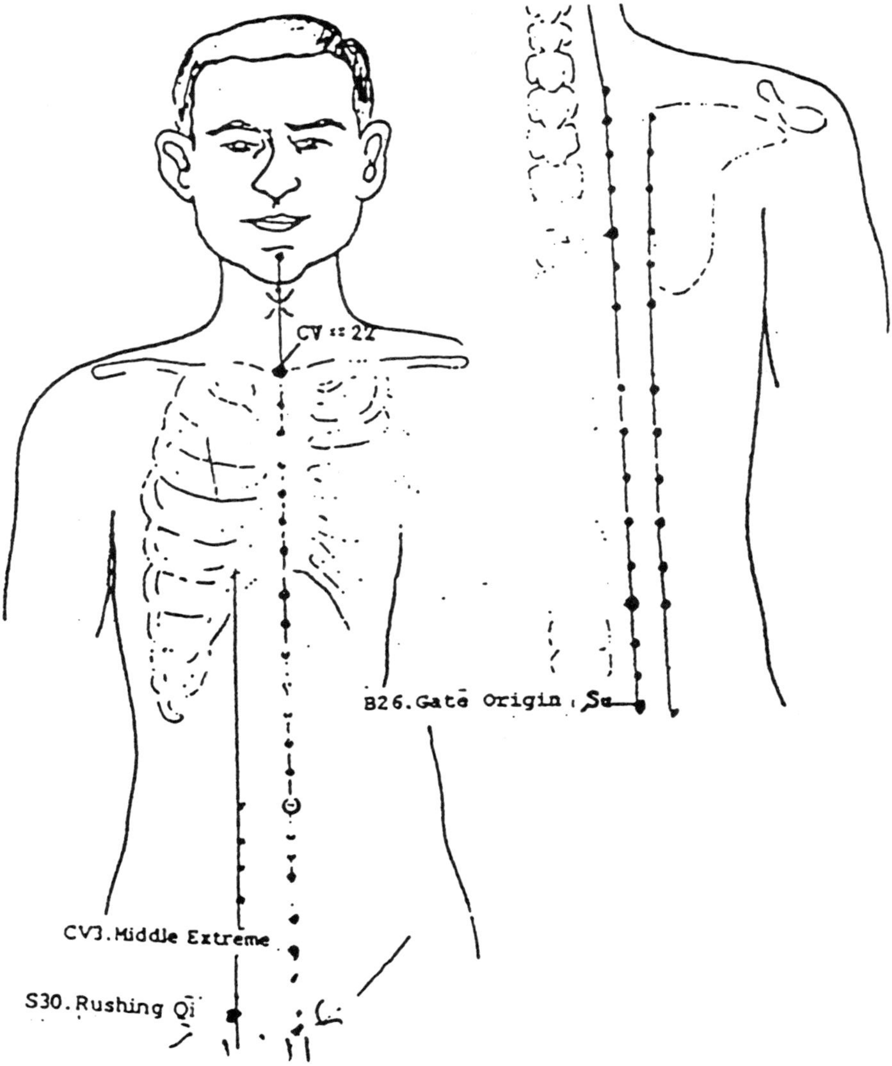

FIGURE- F30

8. MENSTRUAL IRREGULARITY

The patient has pricking pain at the center of the lower abdomen prior to menstruation or during the menstruation period. When the ailment is serious, it would produce dizziness, headache, nausea, pain at loins and legs, etc.

The following Acupunctural points are for treatment, as illustrated in Figure F.31.

a. Point B26Gate Origin Su

Location: See the Section on Large Intestine Catarrh.

b. Point CV.6Sea of Qi.

Location: Two inches below the naval.

Depth of Insertion: For the point B26, seven tenths to eight tenths of an inch in depth. For the point Cv.6,one inch to one and three tenths of an inch.

Treatment: Have the patient lying flat on his back. Insert the needle downward and when it reaches the proper depth and its resonance is felt at the afflicted area under the uterus, provide some stimulation for two or three minutes before extracting the needle. When the resonance is not produced at the desired area,try to seek the right point for the needle insertion until the resonance is produced. If the pain is not relieved by one treatment, repeat two or three more similar treatments.

Effects: Usually one or two separate treatments would bring about the desirable effect.

Note: Those patients with habitually irregular menstruation should receive treatments a few days prior to the beginning of menstruation--providing one treatment every day for two or three days. If the similar treatments are administered for two or three months, this ailment should be completely cured.

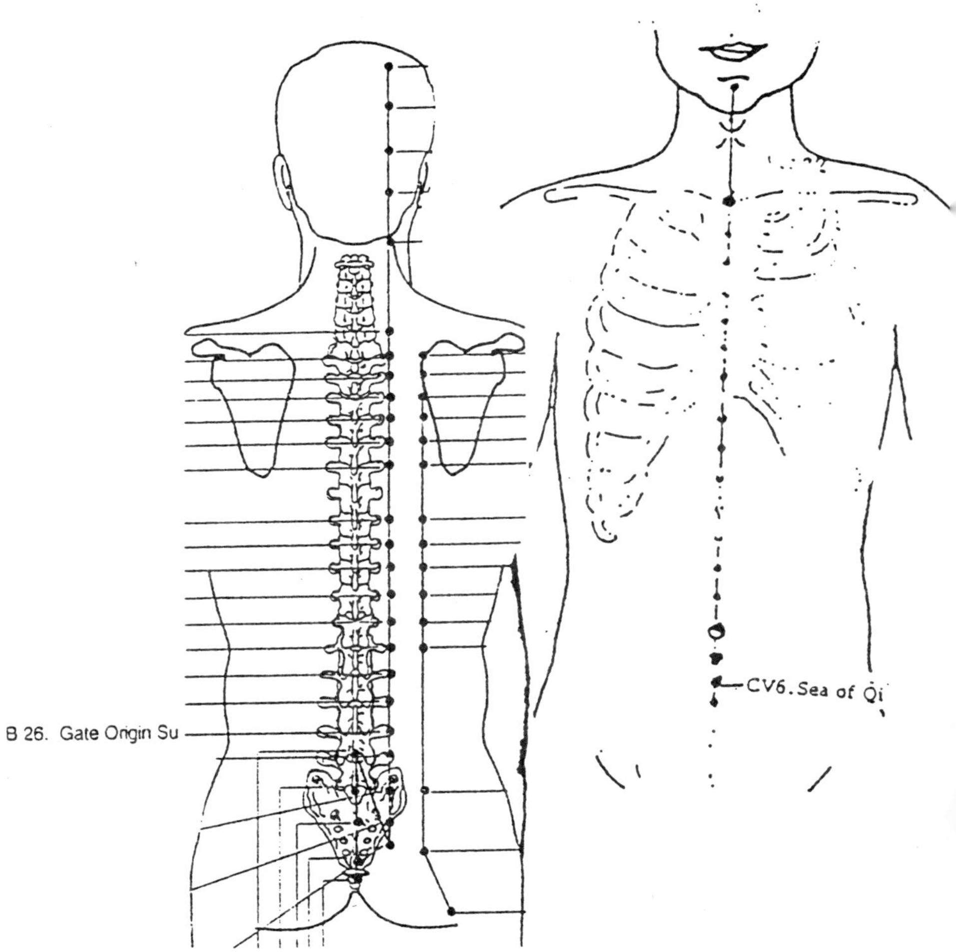

FIGURE- F31

9. THE PELVIS INFLAMMATION

The symptoms are similar to those for lumbago. The difference is in the pelvic inflammation resulting from the inflamed genital organs or inflammation around these organs, which cause an irregularity in menstruation and other pains.

The recommended Acupunctural points ar as follows(see Figure F.32):

a. Point CV.3Middle Extreme.

   Location: See the Section on Bladder Caterrh.

b. Point S30Rushing Qi.

   Location: Two inches off from the center line in the lower abdomen, just below where one can feel the pulse of the femoral artery.

c. Point SP.6Three Yin Crossing.

   Location: Four inches above the inside of each ankle-bones.

d. Point B26Gate Origin Su.

   Location: One fifth of an inch from the center line under the lumbar vertebra on each side.

e. Points S36Leg Three Miles and LI.11 Crooked Pond.

   Location: See the Section on Large Intestine Catarrh.

Depth of Insertion: One half to seven tenths

of an inch in depth.

<u>Treatment</u>: The patient's position--lying flat on his back with his arms and legs out stretched. Insert the needle but barely touching the tibia bone. When the needle reaches the proper depth and its resonance is felt around the toes, provide some tapping stimulation for thirty seconds before pulling the needle out.

<u>Effects</u>: When the ailments is mild, three or four separate treatments--once in every other day--should be enough to produce good results. When the ailment is serious, several treatments--given consecutively every day--are required to produce good results.

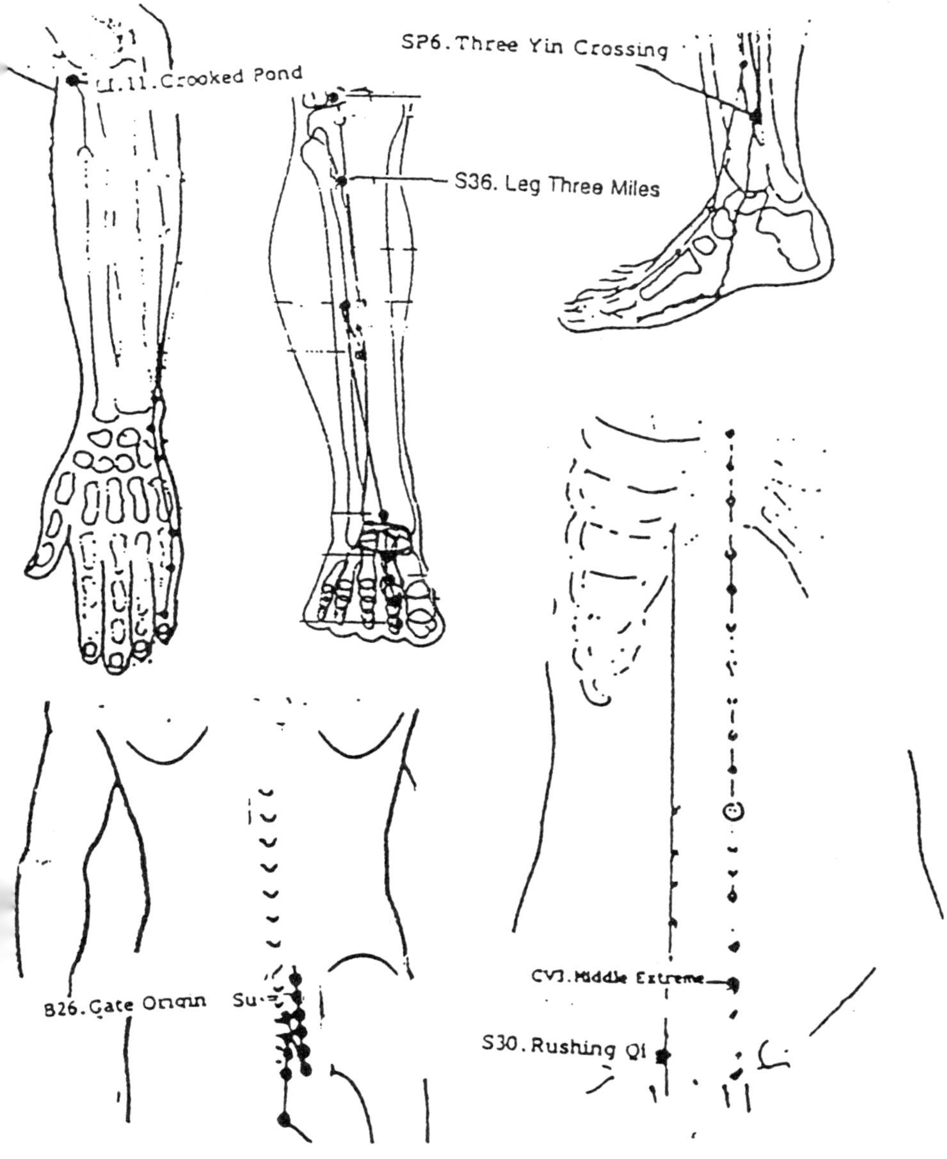
LI.11.Crooked Pond
SP6.Three Yin Crossing
S36. Leg Three Miles
B26.Gate Origin
CV3.Middle Extreme
S30.Rushing Qi

FIGURE- F32

10. LUMBAGO

The patient feels pain on one side or both sides of fifth lumbar vertebra. The patient experiences difficulty to move about his waist, such as bending, sitting,k or turning his body.

The following are the Acupunctural points to be treated, as shown in Figure F.33.

a. Point B26Gate Origin Su.

Location; See the Section on Large Intestine Catarrh.

b. Other points:CV.12Middle Channel,GV.14 Big Hammer,B25Large Intestine Su,and CV.13Middle Extreme.

Depth of Insertion: Seven tenths to eight tenths of an inch.

Treatment: The treatment difference between lumbago and large intestine catarrh is that a stronger stimulation of the needle is required for the former than for the latter. Accordingly, it would be effective by providing some intermediate degree of stimulation for several minutes and by repeating the same treatment a few more times.

Effects: Mild symptoms of this ailment can be cured by two successive treatments. The chronic ones can be cured by several treatments--providing once in every once in every other day.

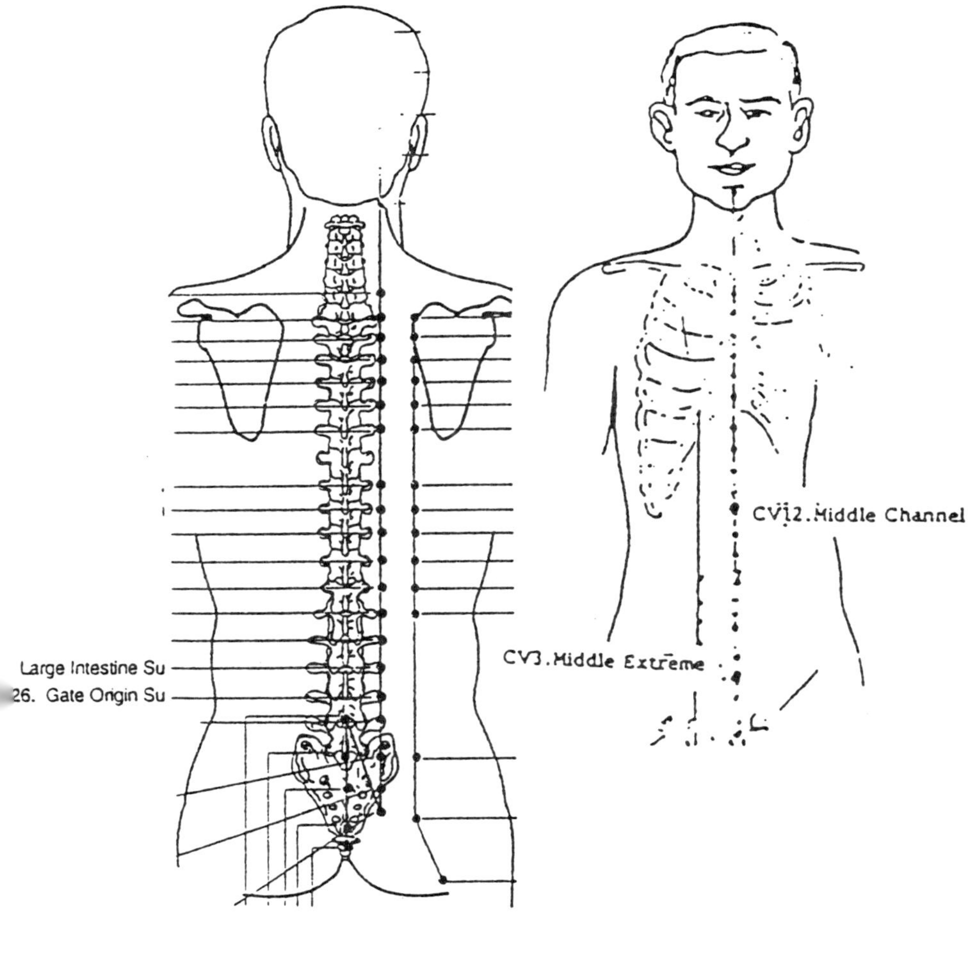

Large Intestine Su
26. Gate Origin Su
CV12. Middle Channel
CV3. Middle Extreme

FIGURE - F 33

PSALM 118:22

THE STONE WHICH THE BUILDERS REFUSED IS BECOME THE HEAD STONE OF THE CORNER.

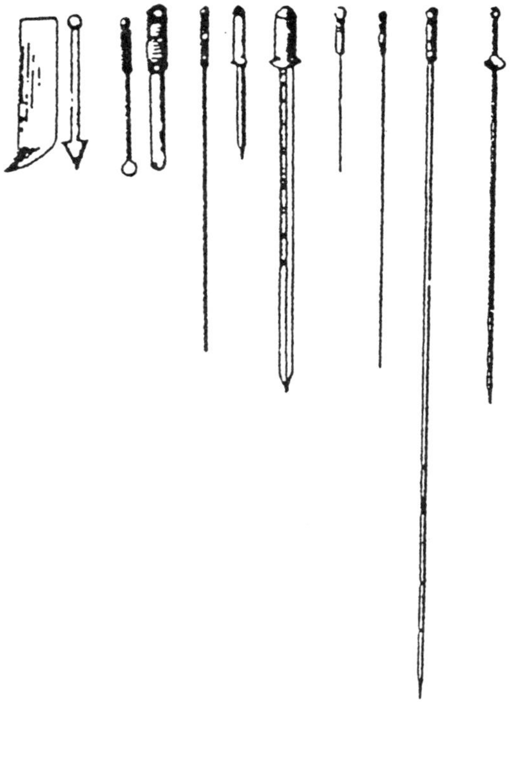

- NEEDLES -

CHAPTER VII

AILMENTS OF LOWER LIMBS

CHAPTER VII
AILMENTS OF LOWER LIMBS

1. CHRONIC KNEE ARTHRITIS

The following are some of the symptoms:when walking, climbing the stairs, sitting, or standing up from the sitting position, the knees ache, or cause the feeling of icy coldness.

The Acupunctural points for treatment are as follows(See Figure F.34):

a. Point S34Bean Mound.

Location:a little above the patella.

b. Point B54Commanding Middle.

Location: This point is located at the center of the hollow inside of the knee. It is treated for both acute pain and icy coldness in the knees.

c. Other commonly applied points: LV8 Crooked Spring,S36Leg Three Miles,GB34 Yang Mound Spring,andSP10Sea of Blood.

Depth of Insertion: One half to three fifths of an inch for both points, S34 and B54.

Treatment: The patient's position: Lying flat on his back. For the treatment of the point S34,insert the needle straight down into the skin, and when it reaches the proper depth and its resonance is felt at the afflicted area, stop any further insertion and provide some stimulation for two or three minutes(Don not extract the needle yet). Push the needle one tenth of an inch deeper and provide some more stimulation for two or three minutes before extracting the needle. The resonant treatment would alleviate the pain.

For the treatment of the point BBB, the needle insertion should follow the same procedure as in the case of the point S34. In treating this point, one should continuously watch for the resonance to reach the afflicted area, where the patient feels icy coldness.

Effects: Four or five separate treatments--once in every other day--should suffice to bring about good results.

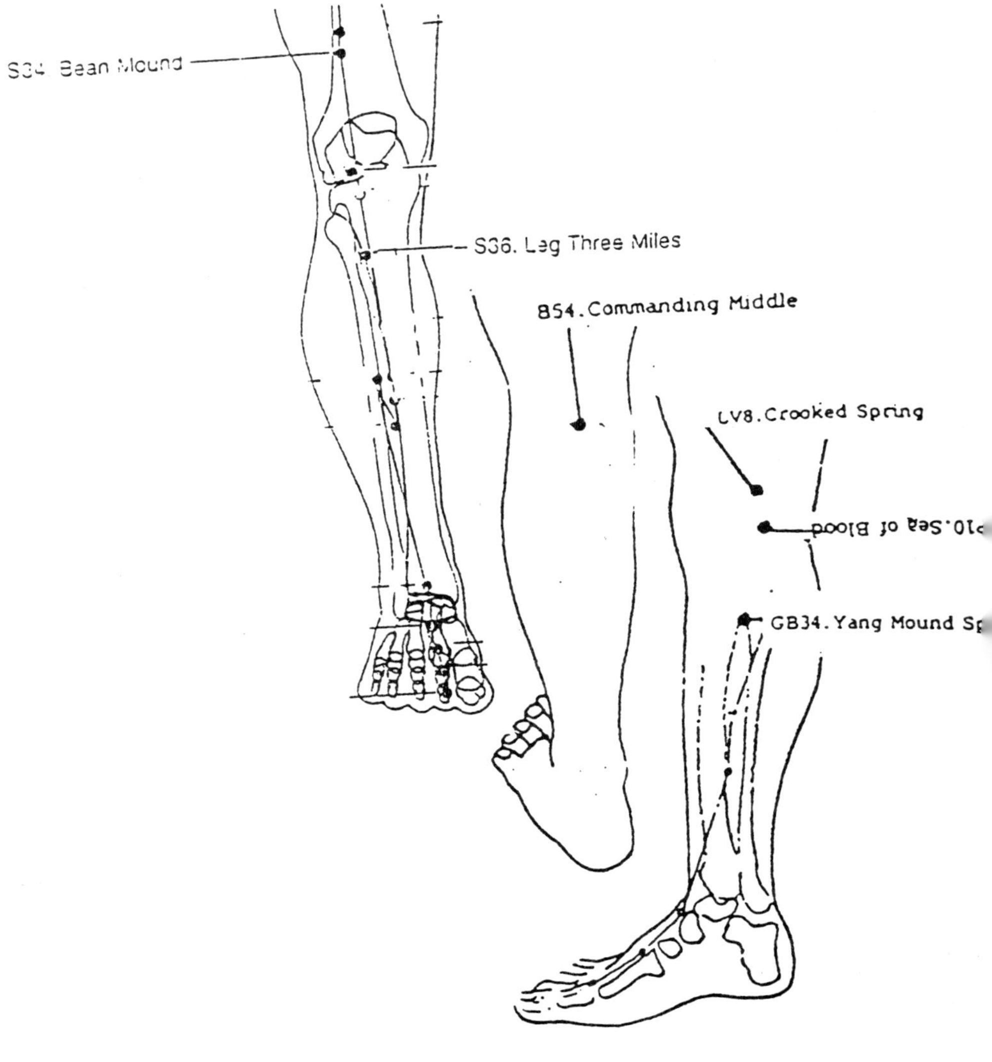
S34. Bean Mound
S36. Leg Three Miles
B54. Commanding Middle
LV8. Crooked Spring
GB34. Yang Mound Sp

FIGURE- F34

2. ACUTE ARTHRITIS OF THE KNEE

The knee is swollen and painful. The following are the Acupunctural points to be treated, as shown in Figure F.35:

a. Point S31Thigh Gate.
   Location: This point is situated along side the ilium. In the case of acute arthritis, when one presses on this point, the patient would feel the stimulation all the way to the knee.
b. Points LV.2Colum Inbetween and B54Commanding Middle.

Depth of Insertion: Eight tenths of an inch to one inch in depth.

Treatment: The patient's position--lying flat on his back and letting his legs resting on a pillow. Press the needle vertically into the skin, and when it reaches the proper depth and its resonance is felt at the afflicted area, stop further insertion. Provide some stimulation for two or three minutes and allow the patient to feel the pain being dissipated. Following this, press the needle one tenth of an inch deeper and provide some more stimulation for two or three minutes before extracting the needle. If the patient does not experience the dissipation of pain, then repeat the above treatment by adjusting the point of insertion or the angle of the needle. The dissipation of pain depends upon the intensity of sensation felt at the afflicted area.

Effects: The pain and swelling in the knee can be alleviated by one treatment, and their complete cure can be obtained by three or four separate treatments. The patient with walking difficulty can walk after just one treatment.

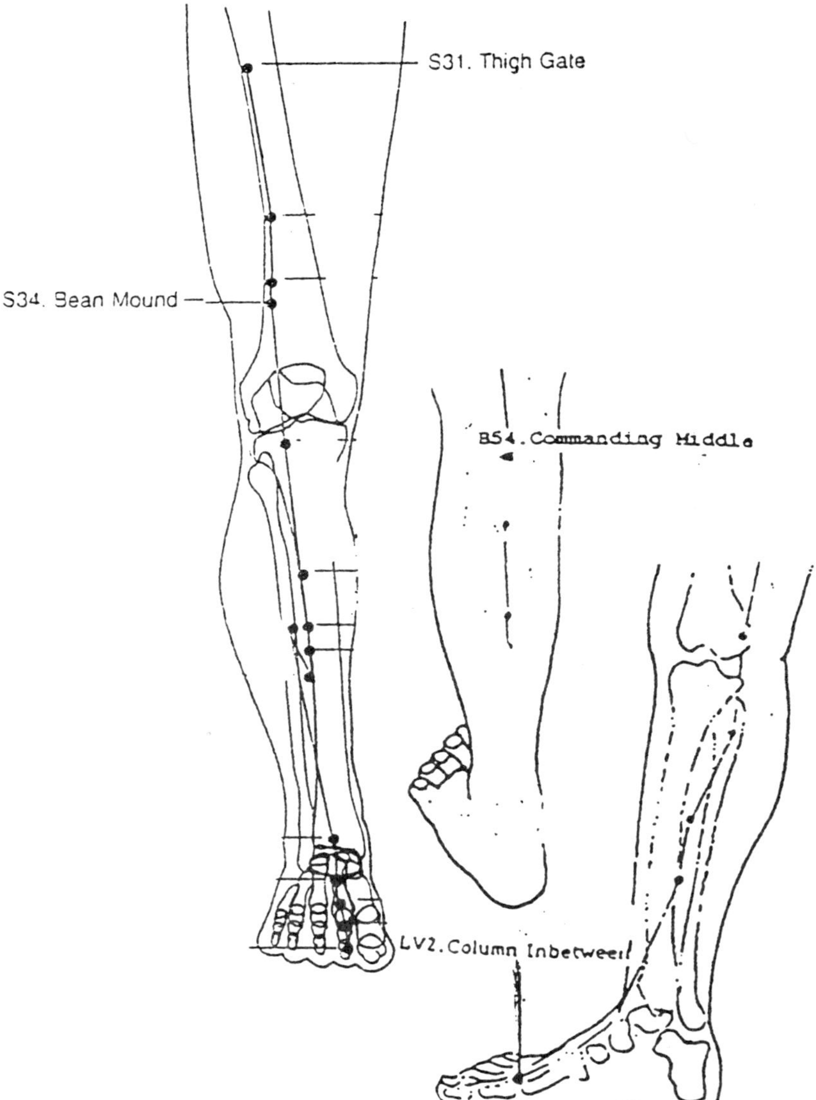
S31. Thigh Gate
S34. Bean Mound
B54. Commanding Middle
LV2. Column Inbetween

FIGURE- F35

3. INFLAMMATION OF BIG TOE

The patient experiences pain or irritation at the first phalanges of the big toe or around it. He would feel pain whenever he attempts to move about the toe or whenever the toe touches the ground while walking.

The Acupunctural point, LV2Colum Inbetween,as shown in Figure F.36, is generally used for treating such an ailment. This point is located between the big toe and the second toe.

Depth of Insertion: One third to three fifths of an inch.

Treatment: Have the patient lying flat on his back. The needle goes into the skin beside the first metatarsal bone. In the case of acute ailment, stop the needle insertion at the depth of one third of an inch and provide mild stimulation for one minute. Then, push the needle one tenth of an inch deeper and provide some more stimulation before extracting the needle. The inflamed big toe would be significantly relieved right after the first treatment.

The second and third treatment follow the same procedure at the same Acupunctural point, and these treatments would produce additional positive result. In the later case, no feeling of resonance is given to the afflicted area.

In a chronic case, insert the needle into the proper depth and when its resonance reaches the afflicted area, provide some stimulation for one minute before pulling the needle out. It is important that a feeling or sensation should be experienced in the cases of chronic ailment in contrast to those of acute ailment.

When the needle point touches the edge of the first metatarsal bone, the feeling of resonance would easily reach the afflicted area.

Effects: Acute inflammation of the big toe can be cured by two or three successive treatments. Chronic cases can be cured by four or five treatments--given once in every other day.

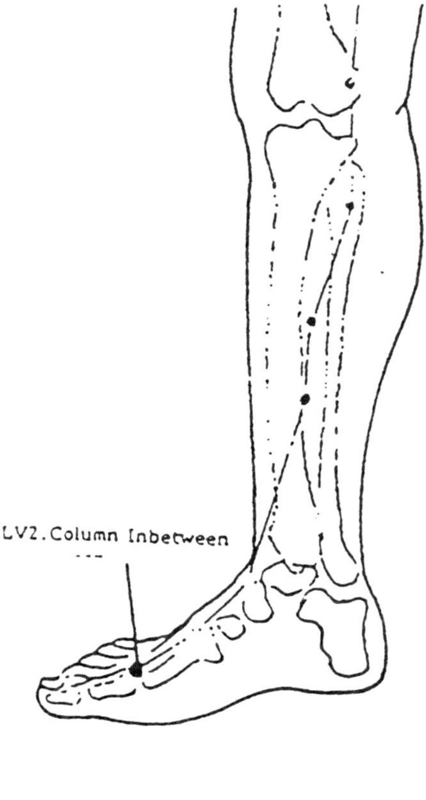

FIGURE- F36

4. <u>CHRONIC ARTHRITIS AT FEMUR JOINTS</u>

Whenever the patient attempts to walk or move his legs, he would feel pain at the head of the femur bone. He would often feel heat or irritation inside the joints. For such an ailment, the Acupunctural point GB.30Jumping Circle in Figure F.37 is used for its treatment. This point is located at the outside of the femur bone head, where there is a hollow spot beside the edge of the gluteus maximus muscle.

Depth of Insertion: Eight tenths of an inch to one inch in depth.

Treatment: Have the patient lying on his side with his legs bend at 120 degree. Insert the needle vertically into the skin and when the needle reaches the required depth and its resonance is felt at the afflicted area, stop any further insertion. Provide some tapping stimulus for three or four minutes. Again, press the needle one or two tenths of an inch deeper and provide some more tapping stimulus for three or four minutes before extracting the needle.The needle feeling reaches the aching area, and the patient would experience a comfortable feeling.

For further effect, repeat the similar treatment two or three more times. In the case of some patients having acute arthritis and feeling a burning pain in the afflicted area, the procedure for needle insertion and its depth would be different.In such cases,insert the needle with mild tapping into the depth of one third to two fifths of an inch. Provide some tapping stimulus for thirty seconds before pulling the needle out. It is noted here that it is better not to produce any feeling from the needle. Insert five or six needles around the main point GB.30 in Figure F.37, thereby completing the first treatment. After two or three separate treatments like this one, the acuteness of the ailment would dissipate. As for the chronic type of ailments, similar treatments should be administered.

Effects: Two or three treatments are required to relieve any acute type of ailments. However, three to six treatments are required for any chronic type.

Note: In addition to the point GB.20, other commonly used points are GB.28Binding Path,S34 Bean Mound,S32Prostrate Hare,SP.11Basket Door, and LV.10Five Miles,as illustrated in Figure F.37.

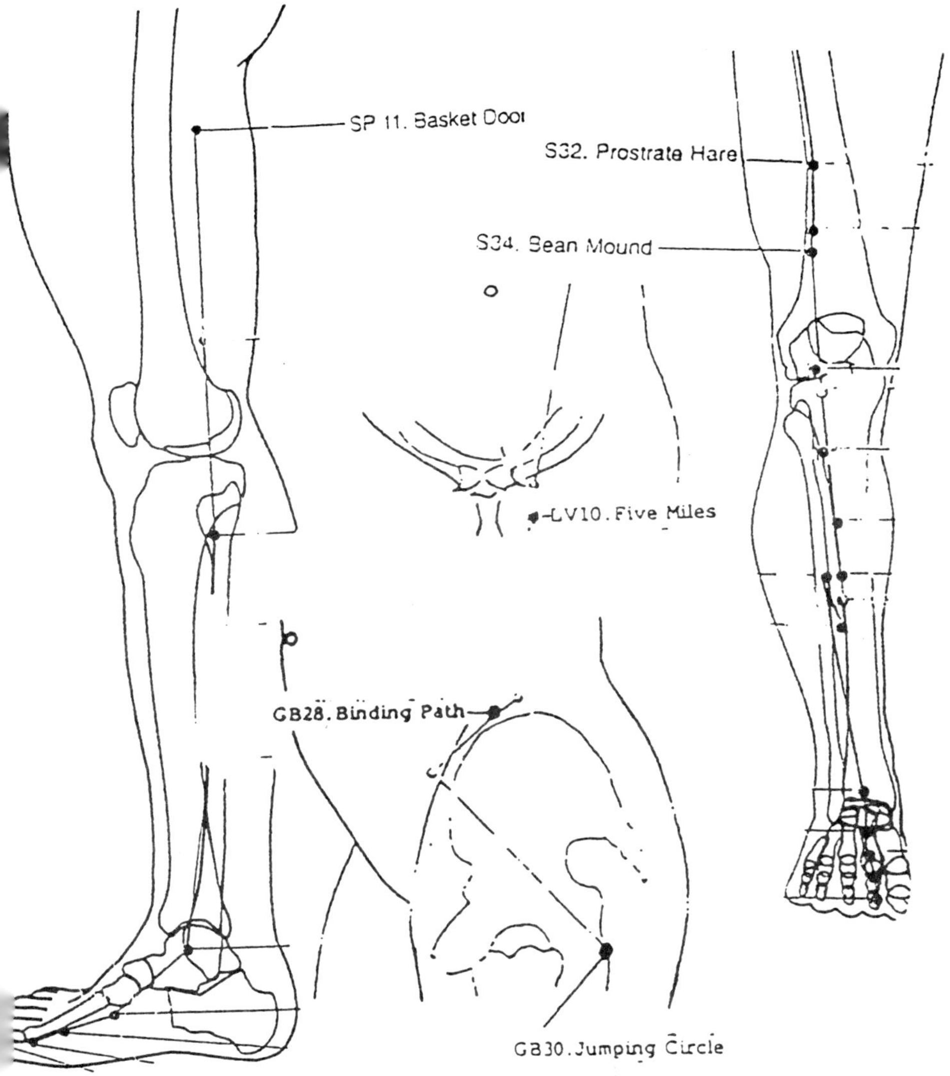
SP 11. Basket Door
S32. Prostrate Hare
S34. Bean Mound
LV10. Five Miles
GB28. Binding Path
GB30. Jumping Circle

FIGURE - F37

5. SCIATICA

Patients would experience acute dull pain along the nerve channel at the hip and throughout the back of thigh and leg.

The following Acupunctural points are recommended for treatment, as shown in Figure F 38.

a. Point GB.30Jumping Circle Rear.

Location: Behind the femur head between the gluteus maximus and gluteus medius.

b. Point B51Prosperous Gate.

Location: Six inches below the ischium joints on the back of thigh.

c. Point B55Uniting Yang.

Location: Two inches below the knee on the rear side of the leg.

d. Point GB.36Outer Mound.

Location: Seven inches from the lateral malleolus in front of the fibula.

e. Other points: B23KIdney Su and S36Leg Three Miles.

Which of the two points B55 and GB36 is used depends upon where the pain is felt. If the pain is felt around the rear part of the leg, the point B55 should be treated, whereas if the pain is felt around the front part of the leg, the point GB.36 should be treated.

Depth of Insertion: For the point GB.30 Rear--four fifths of an inch to one inch in depth.
For the point B51-----Three fifths to four fifths of an inch.
For the point B55 ------one half to three fifths of an inch.
For the point GB.36-----one half to three fifths of an inch.

Treatment: The patient's position--lying on his stomach with the upper part of his body up and supported by his elbows while his forehead resting on his arms which are folded. For the treatment of the point GB.30, insert the needle toward the ischium. When the needle reaches the proper depth and its resonance goes to the leg through the ischium nerve channel, stop any further insertion and provide some stimulation for one or two minutes. Subsequently, slightly increase the stimulation at the same depth in order to increase the needle resonance before extracting the needle. Care must be taken not to give excessive stimulation to the needle; otherwise, this may cause a sudden dizziness or negative feeling on the part of patient.
For the treatment of the point GB.36, the needle insertion may be made in the same manner as in the above, but the needle point should be aimed toward the fibula in order to produce a feeling of sensation around the fifth toe.

Effects: Newly developed ailment of this kind can be cured or alleviated by two or three treatments--given once every day. For the required--given once every day or every other day.

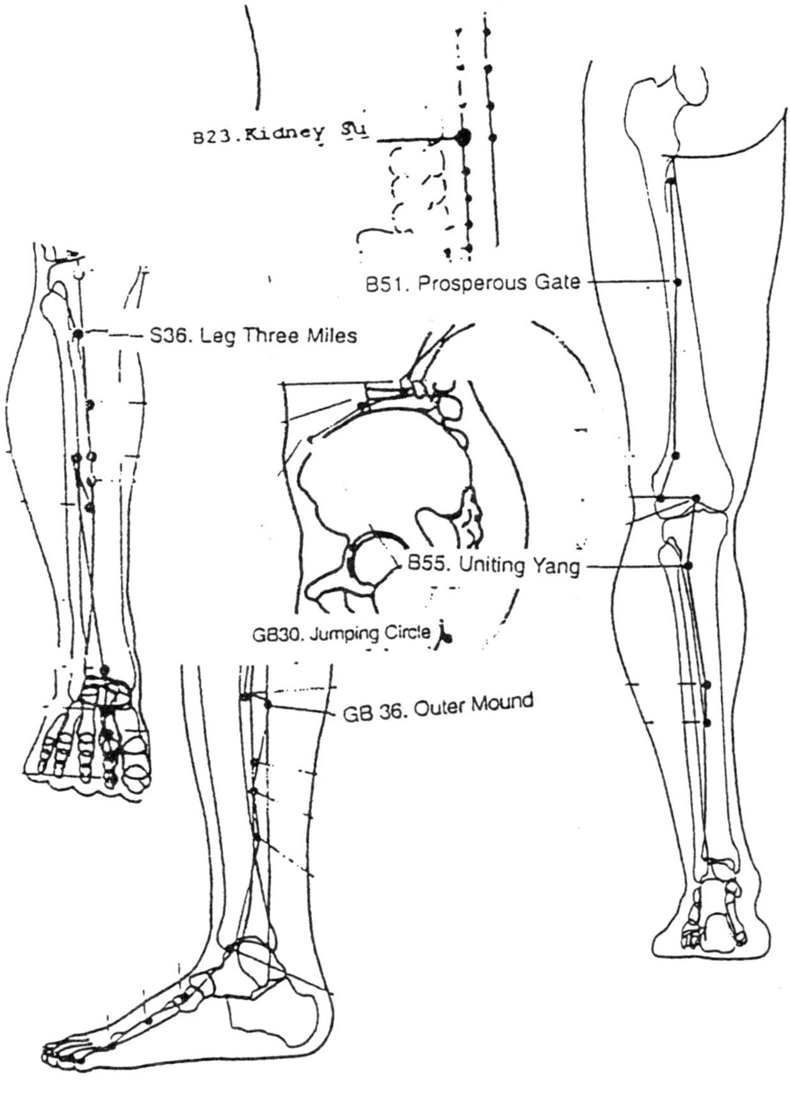
B23. Kidney Su
B51. Prosperous Gate
S36. Leg Three Miles
B55. Uniting Yang
GB30. Jumping Circle
GB 36. Outer Mound

FIGURE- F38

CHAPTER VIII

ACUPUNCTURE ANESTHETICS

CHAPTER VIII
ACUPUNCTURE ANESTHETICS

Ever since the People's Republic of China together with her five thousand year old art of Acupuncture has been "rediscovered", sufficient attention and interest are being aroused among the general public, so that there has evolved some degree of general understanding as to how Acupunctural needles are applied for the purposed of anesthetics. We now come to recognize the fact that no hypnosis, no mystery, and no exaggerated propaganda are involved in the art of Acupuncture and that it has a significant value to the modern medical science.

In this chapter, the author provides a brief explanation of the principle of Acupuncture anesthetics, the instruments used, and the Acupunctural points for anesthesia, which,he hopes, will aid the reader's comprehension of Acupuncture anesthetics.

1. The principle of Acupuncture Anesthetics: The principle of Acupuncture anesthesia or anesthetics i s that of Acupuncture itself. Acupuncture can cure ailments in various parts of the human body while at the same time it can anesthetize these same parts. In short, the principle of Acupuncture may be summarized as follows: The insertion of a needle or needles at certain pertinent points on the surface of the human body and the generation of resonance through the needle stimulation, whereby the stimuli are transmitted through the meridians to the relevant parts of the body, which yield certain effects. In other words, the following principal elements are involved in Acupunctural treatment:First, the Acupunctural insertion points; second, the

depth of stimulation administered through the needles which tend to tonify or soothe the afflicted areas; third, the meridians through which the stimuli travel to certain parts of the body; and finally, the treated parts may be cured or anesthetized. The healing results from stimulation of the needles by twisting or tapping. Care should be exercised to prevent any excessive stimulation. If the stimuli are produced with proper strength and duration, then the anesthetic effect takes place. The most important matter is the accurate selection of the Acupunctural point for insertion, which is associated with the meridians.

2. The Instrument Used for Anesthetics:

a. What kind of needles are used? They are the same needles as used for treating ailments. The most commonly used needle for anesthesia is six centimeters in length. See the pictures in the text.

b. The multipurpose Electro-Therapeutic apparatus used in Acupuncture is "SHOI WEI". This instrument is employed only recently for providing electric stimulation through the needles(instead of tappings by finger) in order to induce anesthesia; thus, the needles are used as conductors. As mentioned in the above, the stimulation induced through the needles should be moderated and lasting. Traditionally, the stimulation was induced by twisting the needles until the operation was performed. Recently, the electric machine was replaced the man power. This instrument produces a battery power of approximately six to eight voltage in the needle and has one second break in the flow of current in every three or four seconds. The voltage and the breaking time can be adjusted depending upon the degree of sensitivity of certain body parts to the stimulus. Se the picture in the text.

3. Selection of Acupunctural Points: It is very crucial to know exactly where the needle insertion is to be made in order to produce the correct anaesthetic effect on a certain part of the human body. As mentioned earlier, the whole system of Acupuncture itself is based on the meridians. Accordingly, one must decide what meridian corresponds to the part or organ of the body under treatment. The points of needle insertion are chosen from the relevant meridians at the distal extremities, such as hands or legs. Certain selected points are used to anesthetize certain parts or organs, such as heart, lungs, stomach, or brain. At the same time, the surface of the body at the point of needle insertion must be anesthetized. For this reason, we choose the meridian which run through the surface of that part of the body to be punctured by Acupuncture--that is, the point in the meridian nearest to the body's part under treatment. At such points, the needles are inserted while maneuvering the needle stimulation. This is in line with the principle involved in Acupuncture. Through the accumulating experiences in the past, the number of needles to be inserted at any given pint have been reduced considerably and the most effective Acupunctural pints have been found; however, there is still much room to develop new knowledge in the field of Acupuncture.

For the sake of illustration, a few examples of what Acupunctural points are employed for certain parts of the human body are given below.

For tooth operations, the pointLI.1Marchant Yang in Figure F.40, which is connected with the large intestinal meridians on both hands, is treated by needle insertion. For painless child-delivery, the point GV.3Yang Gate is treated; this point is located below the fourth lumbar vertebra, while another point is located below the fifth lumber vertebra.

The following are the meridians and the related Acupunctural points for administering local anesthetics on the parts or organs relative to the corresponding meridians. For instance, if the heart is to be anesthetized , the hear meridian and its related point H8Lesser Mansion are chosen for treatment.

MERIDIANS AND RELATED POINTS

Meridians	Points
Large intestine meridian....	LI.1Marchant Yang
Small intestine meridian....	SI.5Yang Valley
Gall bladder meridian.......	GB.15Above
Stomach meridian.........	S36Leg Three Miles
Bladder meridian........	B66Penetrating Valley
Triple warmer meridian.......	T6Branch Ditch
Lung meridian................	L8Meridian Gutter
Heart meridian...............	H8Lesser Mansion

MERIDANS AND RELATED POINTS

Meridians	Points
Liver meridian................	LV.1 Big Heap
Kidney meridian................	K10 Yin Valley
Circle meridian................	P8 Labor Palace
Spleen meridian..........	SP3 Supreme Whiteness

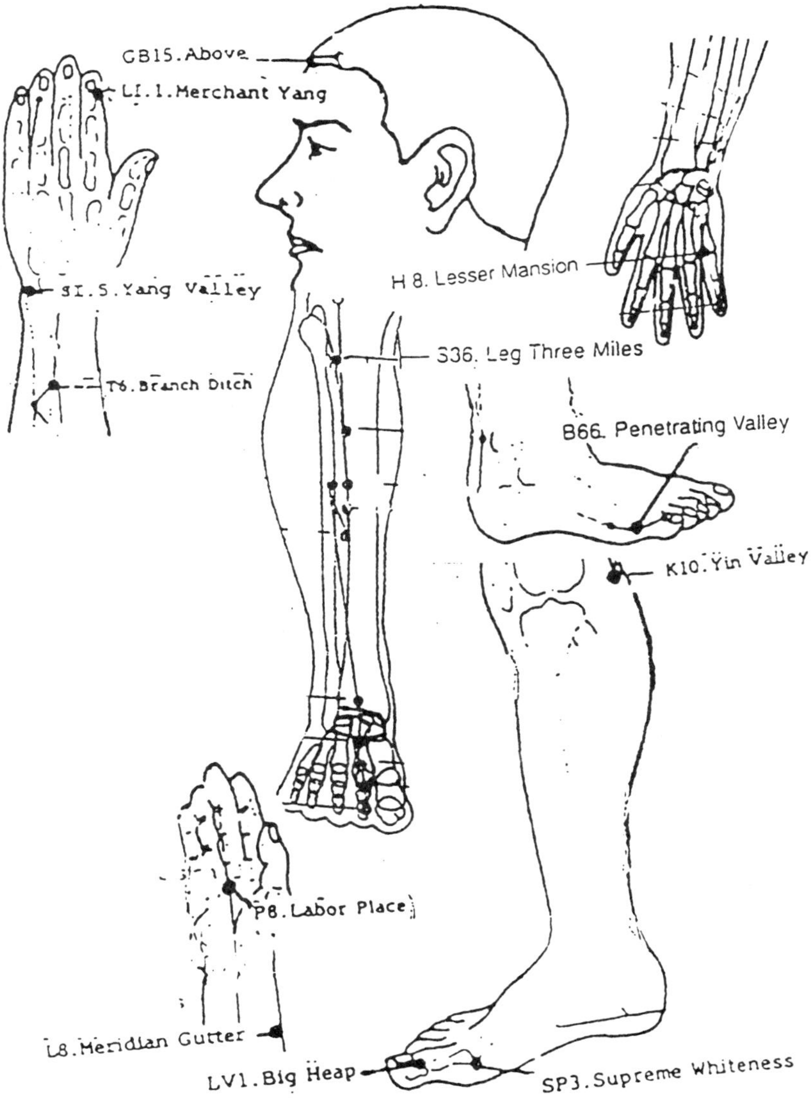
GB15. Above
LI. 1. Merchant Yang
SI. 5. Yang Valley
T6. Branch Ditch
H 8. Lesser Mansion
S36. Leg Three Miles
B66. Penetrating Valley
K10. Yin Valley
P8. Labor Place
L8. Meridian Gutter
LV1. Big Heap
SP3. Supreme Whiteness

FIGURE F40

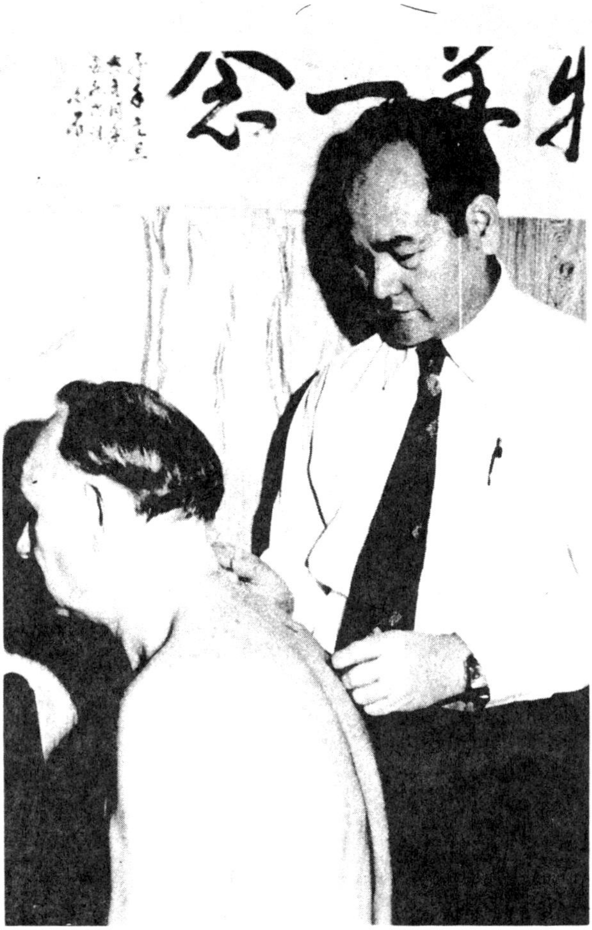

THE AUTHOR GIVING TREATMENT TO A PATIENT WHO HAS A PA

IN THE SHOULDER.

HOW TO USE ACUPUNCTURE NEEDLES

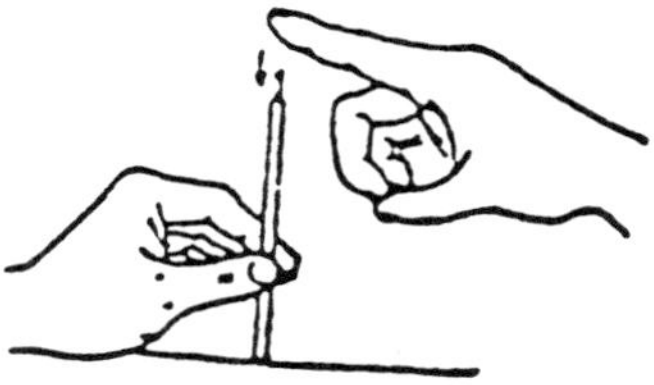

Tubed Acupuncture

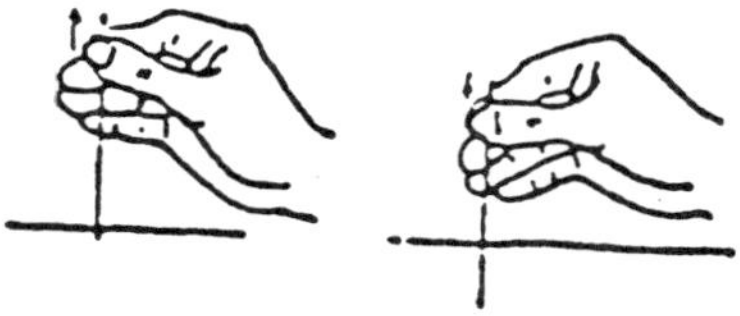

Carry and insert
by hand

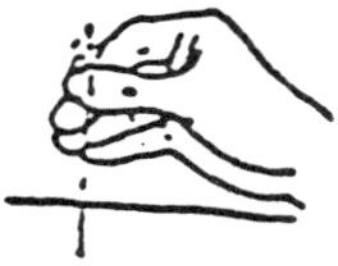

Pushing forward
by thumb

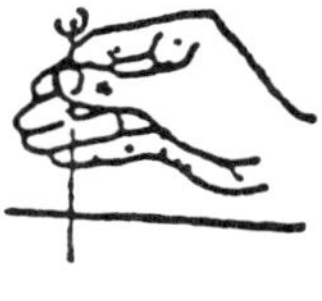

Pullingbackwarad
by thumb

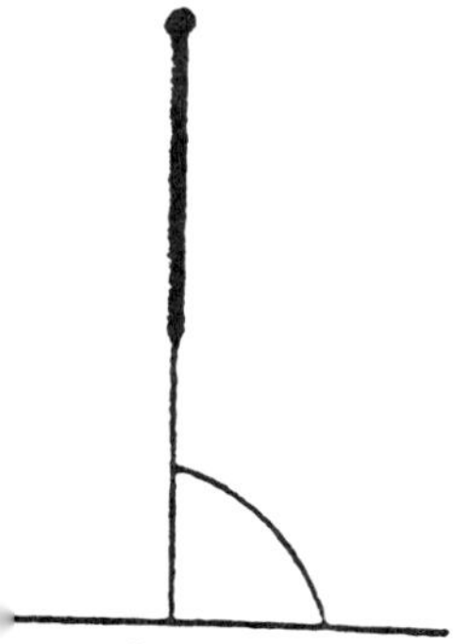

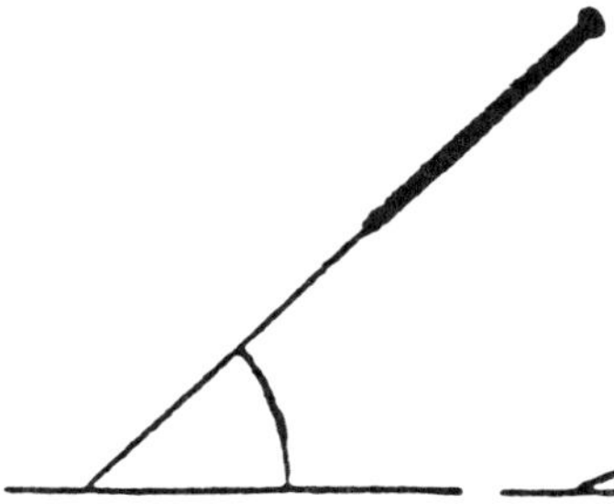

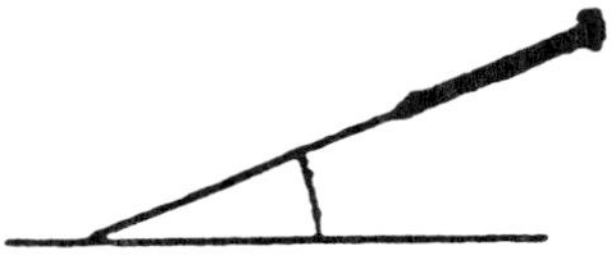

aight piercing

Slant piercing

Horizontal piercing

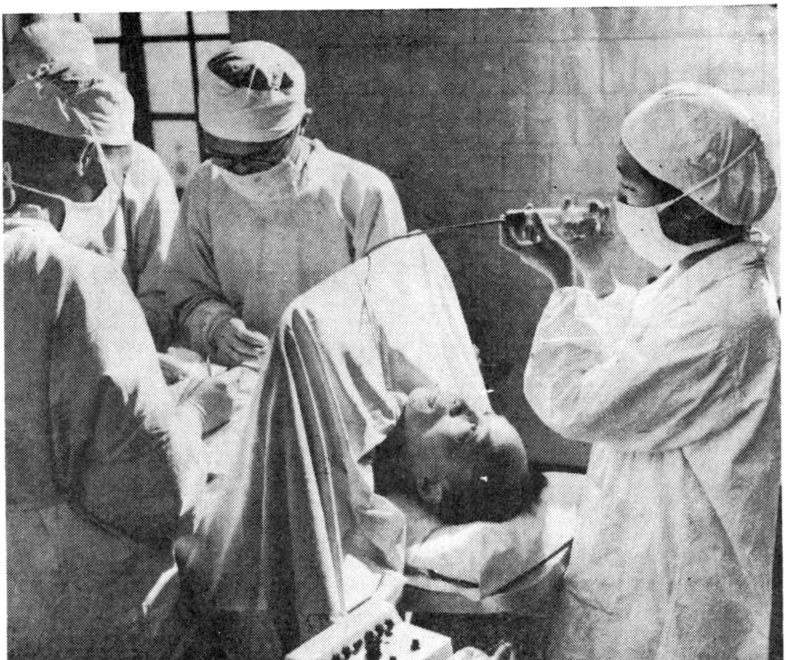

When suturing together of the stomach and intestines is nearly completed, a Chinese herbal brew is introduced into the intestines to stimulate restoration of function.

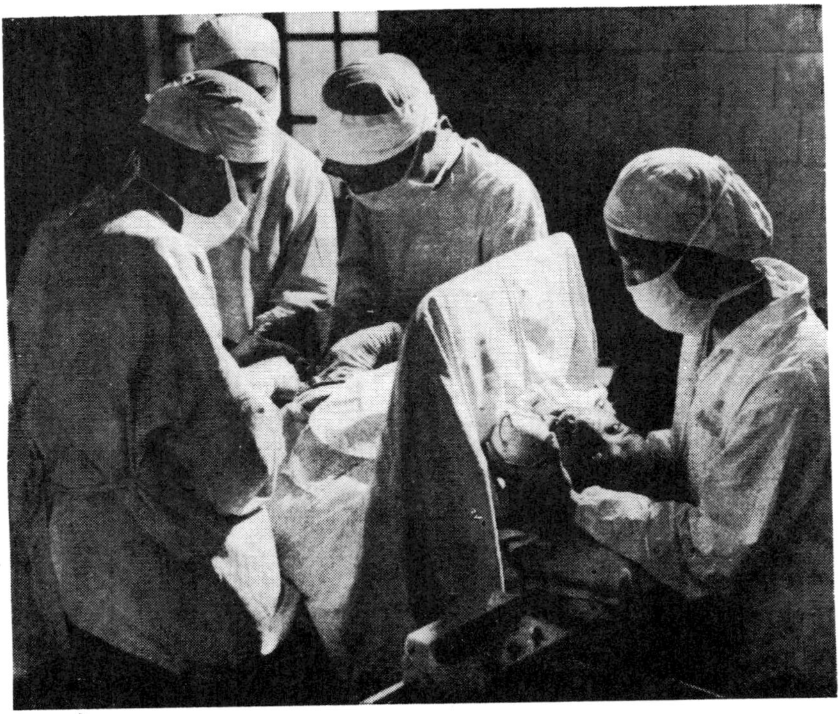

After the rejoining of stomach and intestines is completed, the patient says he is thirsty and is given a drink of water.

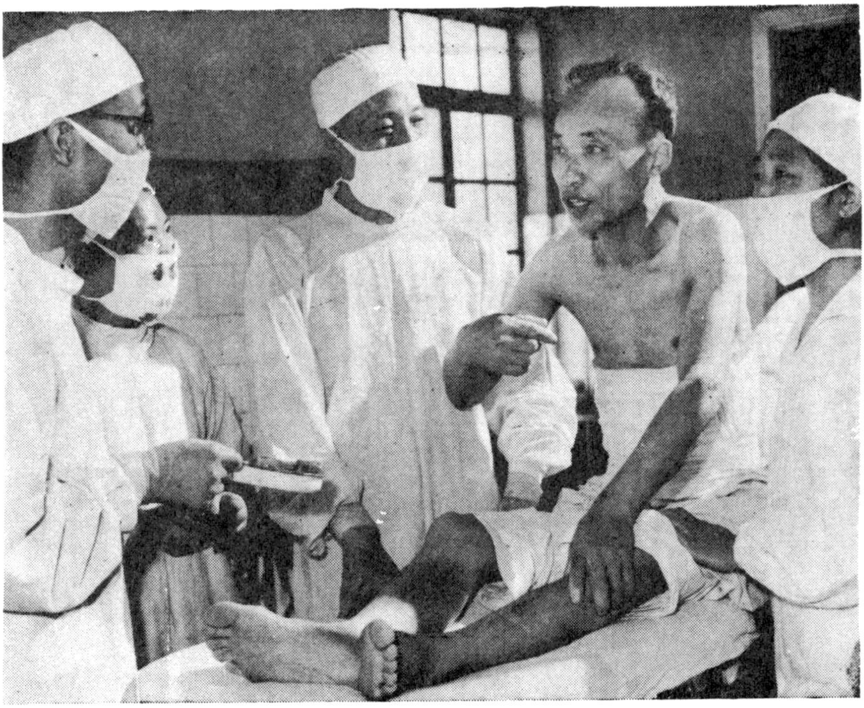

The operation over, the patient sits up and chats with the doctors.

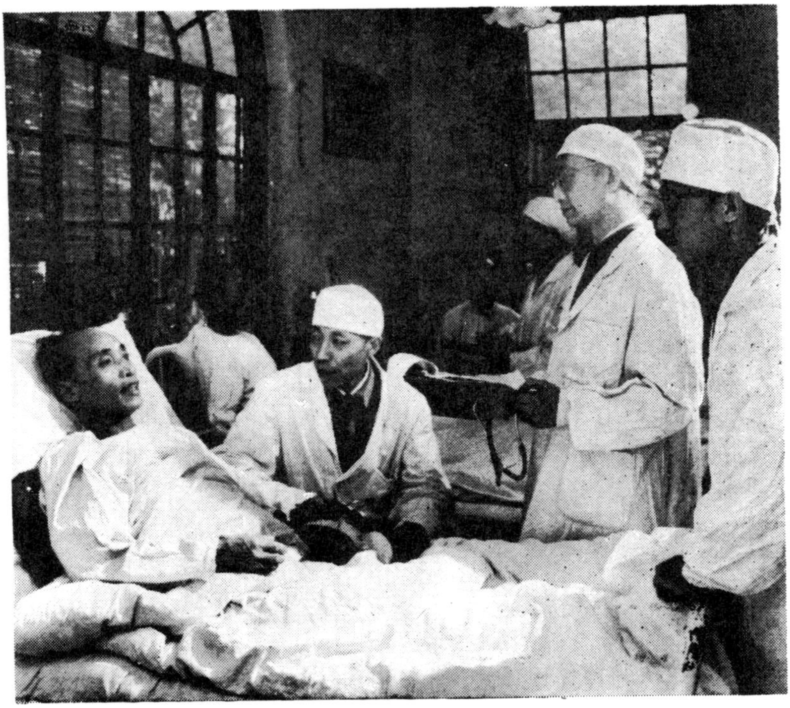

The next day the doctor asks the patient how he felt after taking liquid nourishment orally and the patient says he feels normal.

1. LUNGS L - (☱) Greater Yin

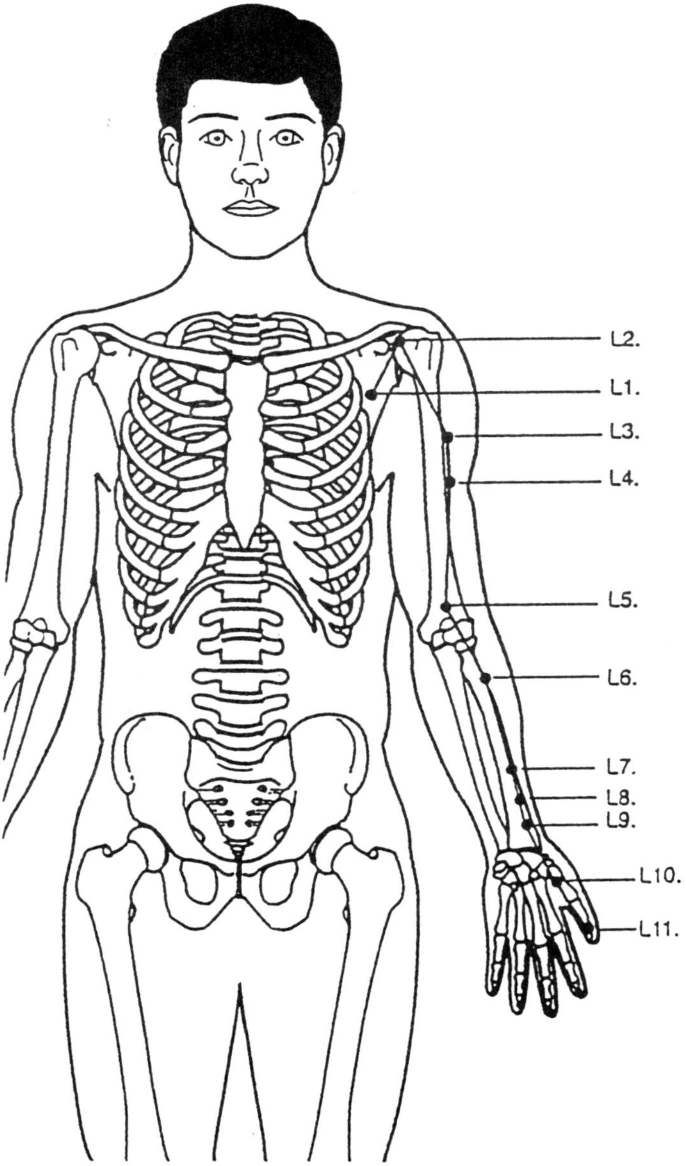

1. Lungs 手太陰肺經 (==)Greater Yin

• —— Impotant Point

代表穴位。

1.	중 부	中府
2.	운 문	雲門
3.	천 부	天府
4.	협 백	俠白
5.	척 택	尺澤 •
6.	공 최	孔最
7.	열 결	列缺 •
8.	경 거	經渠
9.	대 연	大淵 •
10.	어 제	漁際 •
11.	소 상	少商 •

2. LARGE INTESTINE LI - (≡) Sun-Light Yang

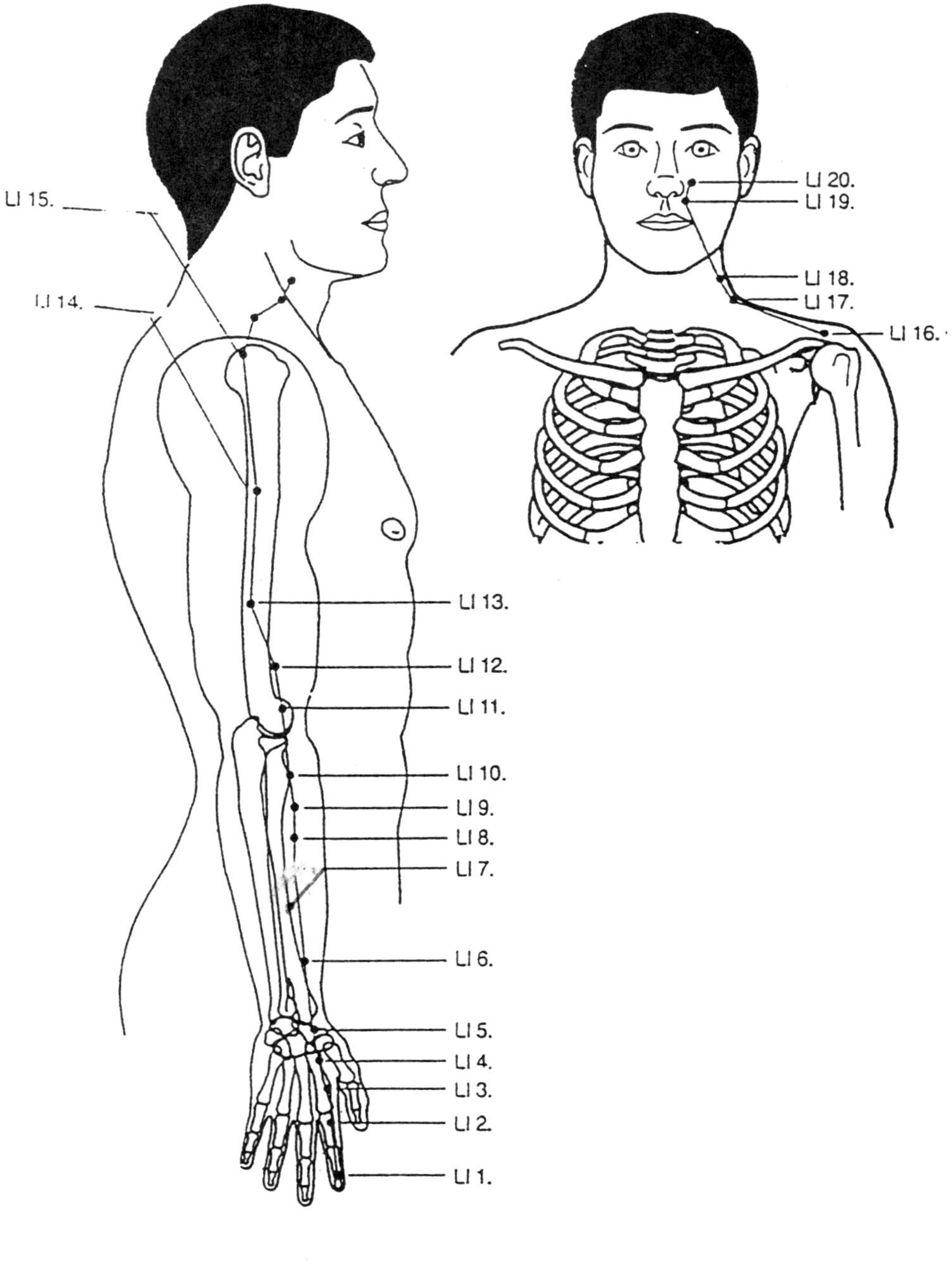

2. Large Intestine 手陽明大腸經 LI(≡)Sun-Light Yang

1. 상	양	商陽 •
2. 이	간	二間
3. 삼	간	三間
4. 합	곡	合谷 •
5. 양	계	陽谿 •
6. 편	역	偏歷 •
7. 온	류	溫溜 •
8. 하	렴	下廉
9. 상	렴	上廉
10. 삼	리	三里
11. 곡	지	曲池 •
12. 주	요	肘髎
13. 오	리	五里
14. 비	노	臂臑
15. 견	우	肩髃 •
16. 거	골	巨骨 •
17. 천	정	天鼎
18. 부	돌	扶突
19. 화	요	禾髎 •
20. 영	향	迎香 •

3. STOMACK S - (☰) Sun-Light Yang

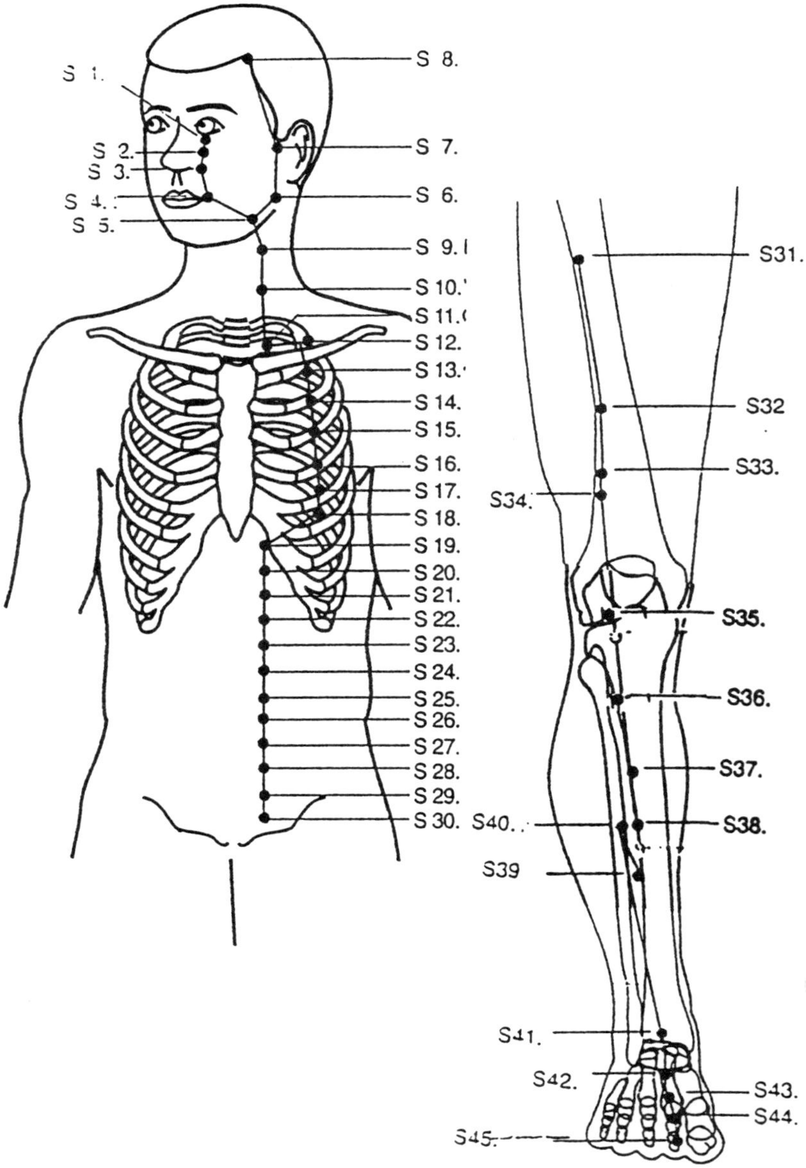

3.Stomach 足陽明胃經 S-(=) Sun-Light Yang

1. 승 읍 承泣
2. 사 백 四白 •
3. 거 료 巨髎 •
4. 지 창 地倉 •
5. 대 영 大迎
6. 협 거 頰車 •
7. 하 관 下關 •
8. 두 유 頭維 •
9. 인 영 人迎
10. 수 돌 水突
11. 기 사 氣舍
12. 결 분 缺盆
13. 기 호 氣戶 •
14. 고 방 庫房
15. 옥 예 屋翳
16. 응 창 膺窓
17. 유 중 乳中
18. 유 근 乳根
19. 불 용 不容
20. 승 만 承滿 •
21. 양 문 梁門 •
22. 관 문 關門
23. 태 을 太乙 •
24. 활육문 滑肉門
25. 천 추 天樞 •
26. 외 릉 外陵
27. 대 거 大巨
28. 수 도 水道
29. 귀 래 歸來 •
30. 기 충 氣衝
31. 비 관 髀關
32. 복 토 伏兎
33. 음 시 陰市 •
34. 양 구 梁丘
35. 독 비 犢鼻 •
36. 삼 리 足三里 •
37. 상 렴 上廉 •
38. 조 구 條口
39. 하 렴 下廉 •
40. 풍 륭 豐隆 •
41. 해 계 解谿 •
42. 충 양 衝陽 •
43. 함 곡 陷谷 •
44. 내 정 內庭 •
45. 여 태 厲兌

4. SPLEEN

SP - (==) Greater Yin

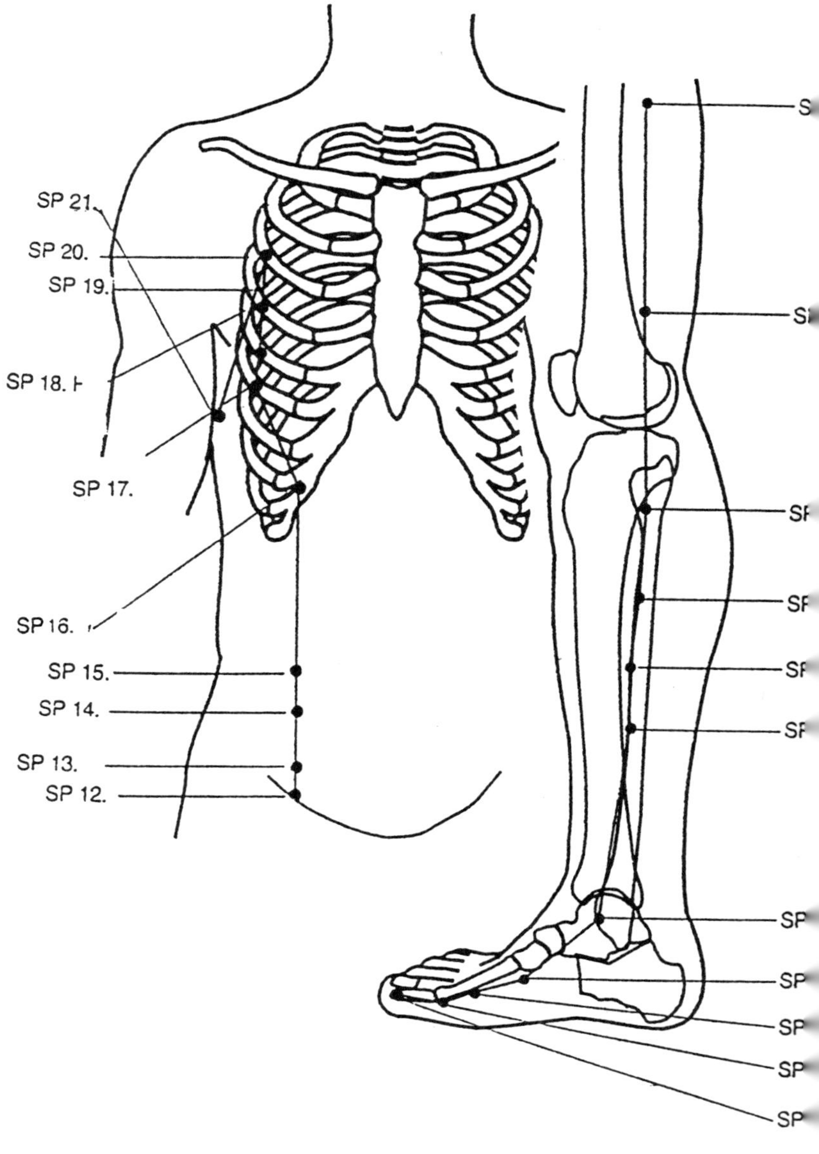

4. Spleen 足太陰脾經 SP- (==) Greater YIN

1.	은 백	隱白	•
2.	대 도	大都	•
3.	태 백	太白	•
4.	공 손	公孫	•
5.	상 구	商丘	•
6.	삼음교	三陰交	•
7.	누 곡	漏谷	•
8.	지 기	地機	•
9.	음릉천	陰陵泉	•
10.	혈 해	血海	•
11.	기 문	箕門	
12.	충 문	衝門	
13.	부 사	府舍	
14.	복 결	腹結	•
15.	대 횡	大橫	
16.	복 애	腹哀	
17.	식 두	食竇	
18.	천 계	天谿	•
19.	흉 향	胸鄕	
20.	주 영	周榮	
21.	대 포	大包	

5. HEART

H - (==) Lesser Yin

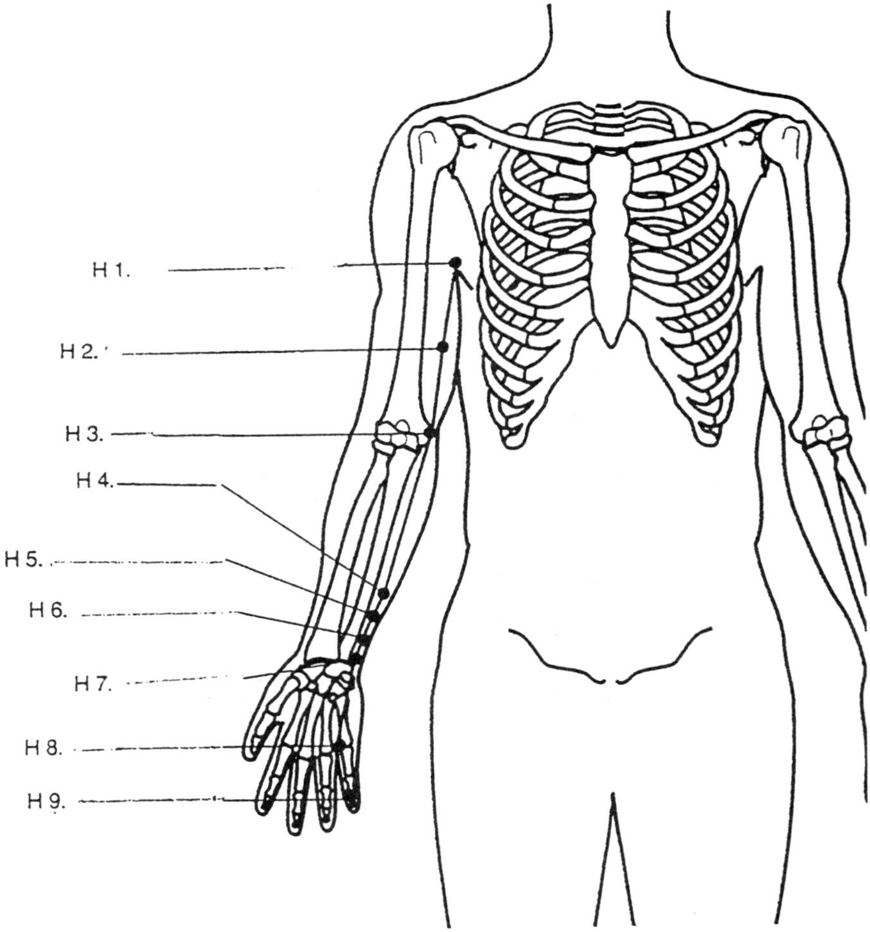

5. HEART 手少陰心經 H - (二) LESSER YIN

1. 극 천 極泉
2. 청 령 靑靈
3. 소 해 少海 •
4. 영 도 靈道
5. 통 리 通里 •
6. 음 극 陰郄 •
7. 신 문 神門 •
8. 소 부 少府 •
9. 소 충 少衝 •

6. SMALL INTESTINE SI - (=) GREATER Yang

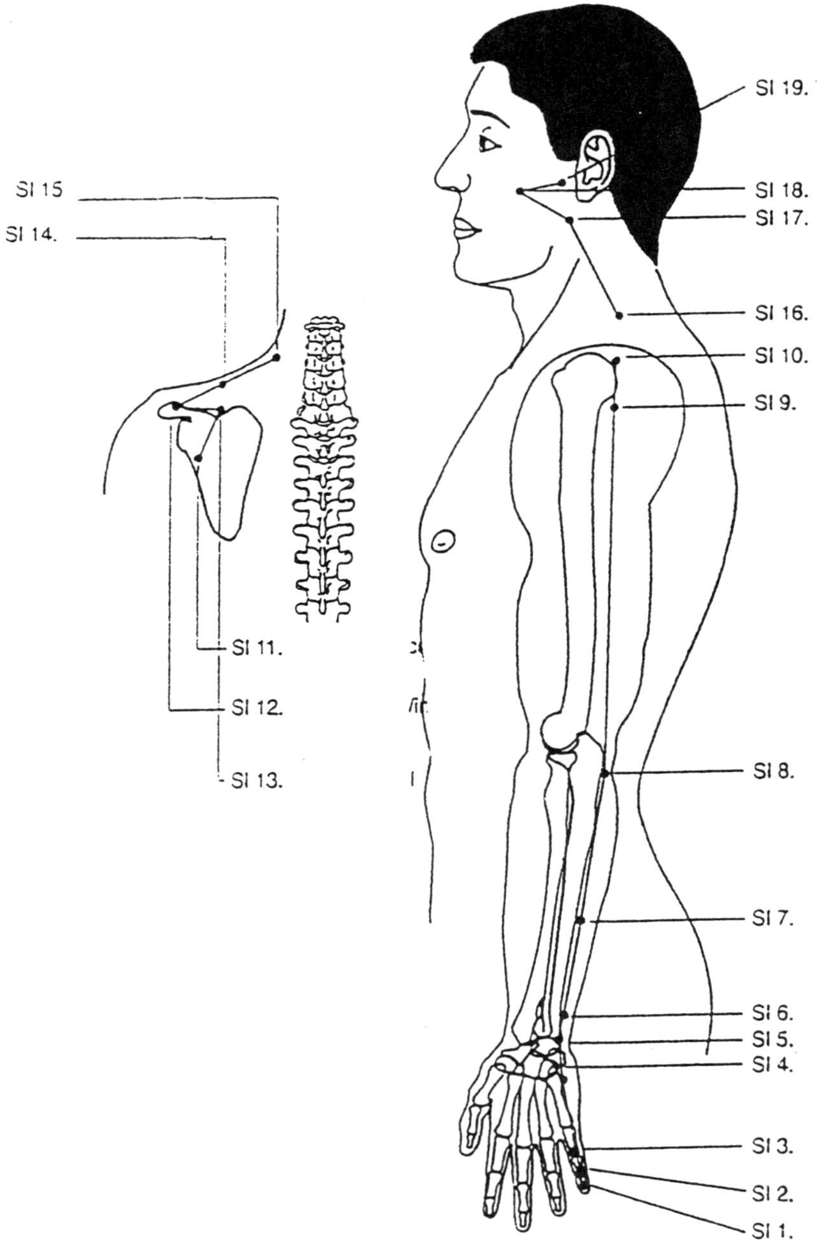

6. Small Intestin 手太陽小腸經 SI-(=) Greater Yang

1. 소 택	少 澤	•
2. 전 곡	前 谷	
3. 후 계	後 谿	•
4. 완 골	腕 骨	•
5. 양 곡	陽 谷	•
6. 양 로	養 老	
7. 지 정	支 正	•
8. 소 해	小 海	
9. 견 정	肩 貞	•
10. 노 유	臑 兪	•
11. 천 종	天 宗	
12. 병 풍	秉 風	
13. 곡 원	曲 垣	•
14. 견외유	肩外兪	•
15. 견중유	肩中兪	•
16. 천 창	天 窓	
17. 천 용	天 容	•
18. 권 료	顴 髎	
19. 청 궁	聽 宮	•

7. BLADDER

B - (=) Greater Yang

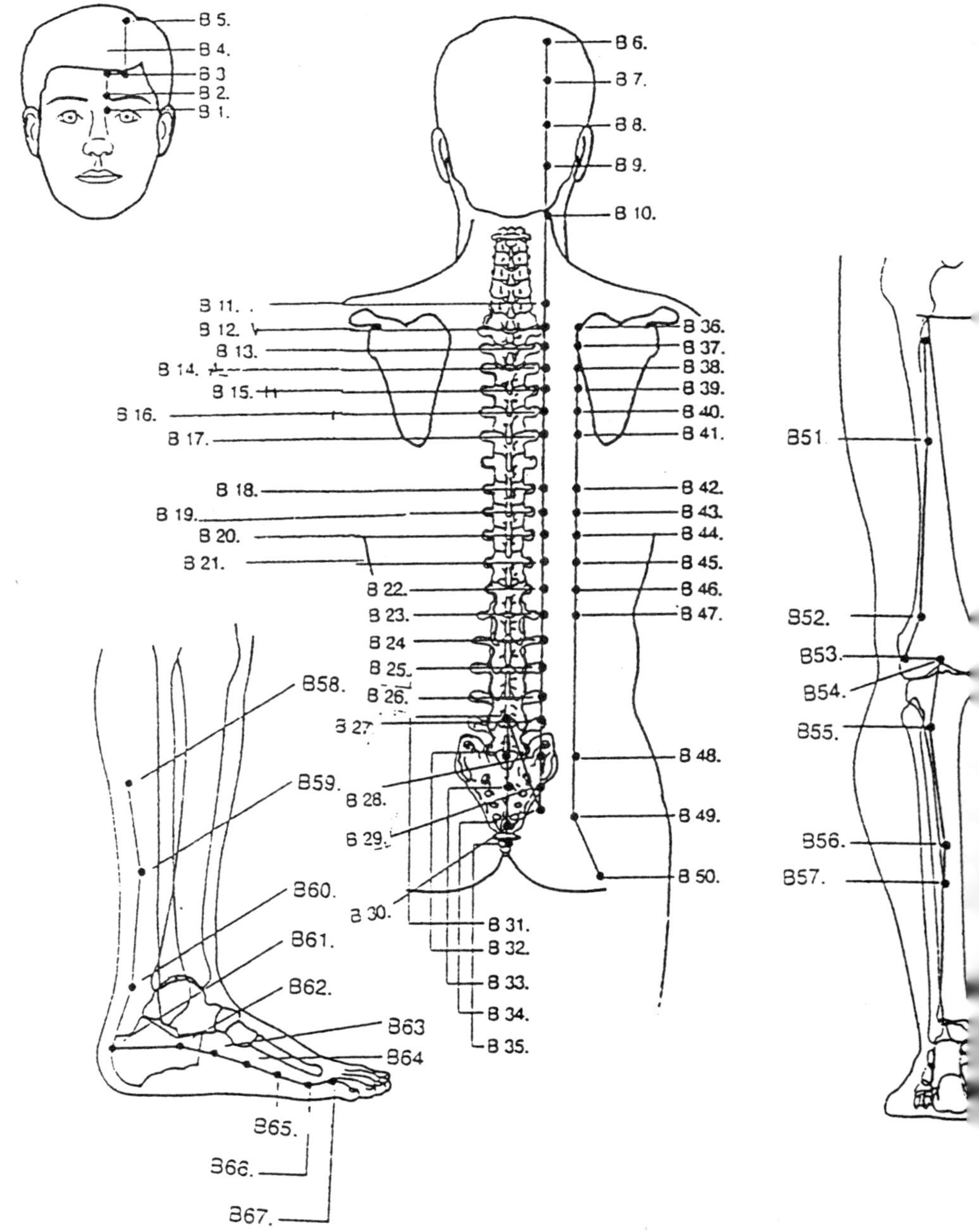

7. BLADDER 足太陽膀胱經 B - (二) GREATER YANG

1. 정명 睛明 •
2. 찬죽 攢竹 •
3. 미충 眉沖
4. 곡차 曲差 •
5. 오처 五處
6. 승광 承光
7. 통천 通天 •
8. 낙각 絡却
9. 옥침 玉枕
10. 천주 天柱 •
11. 대저 大杼
12. 풍문 風門
13. 폐유 肺俞
14. 궐음유 厥陰俞
15. 심유 心俞 •
16. 독유 督俞
17. 격유 膈俞 •
18. 간유 肝俞 •
19. 담유 膽俞
20. 비유 脾俞 •
21. 위유 胃俞 •
22. 삼초유 三焦俞
23. 신유 腎俞 •
24. 기해유 氣海俞
25. 대장유 大腸俞 •
26. 관원유 關元俞
27. 소장유 小腸俞 •
28. 방광유 膀胱俞 •
29. 중려유 中膂俞 •
30. 백환유 白環俞
31. 상료 上髎
32. 차료 次髎 •
33. 중료 中髎
34. 하료 下髎 •
35. 회양 會陽
36. 부분 附分
37. 백호 魄戶
38. 고황 膏肓
39. 신당 神堂
40. 의희 譩譆
41. 격관 膈關 •
42. 혼문 魂門
43. 양강 陽綱
44. 의사 意舍
45. 위창 胃倉 •
46. 황문 肓門
47. 지실 志室 •
48. 포황 胞肓
49. 질변 秩邊
50. 승부 承扶
51. 은문 殷門
52. 부극 浮郄
53. 위양 委陽
54. 위중 委中 •
55. 합양 合陽
56. 승근 承筋 •
57. 승산 承山 •
58. 비양 飛陽
59. 부양 附陽
60. 곤륜 崑崙 •
61. 복삼 僕參
62. 신맥 申脈 •
63. 금문 金門 •
64. 경골 京骨
65. 속골 束骨
66. 통곡 通足 •
67. 지음 至陰 •

8. KIDNEY

K - (☵) Lesser Yin

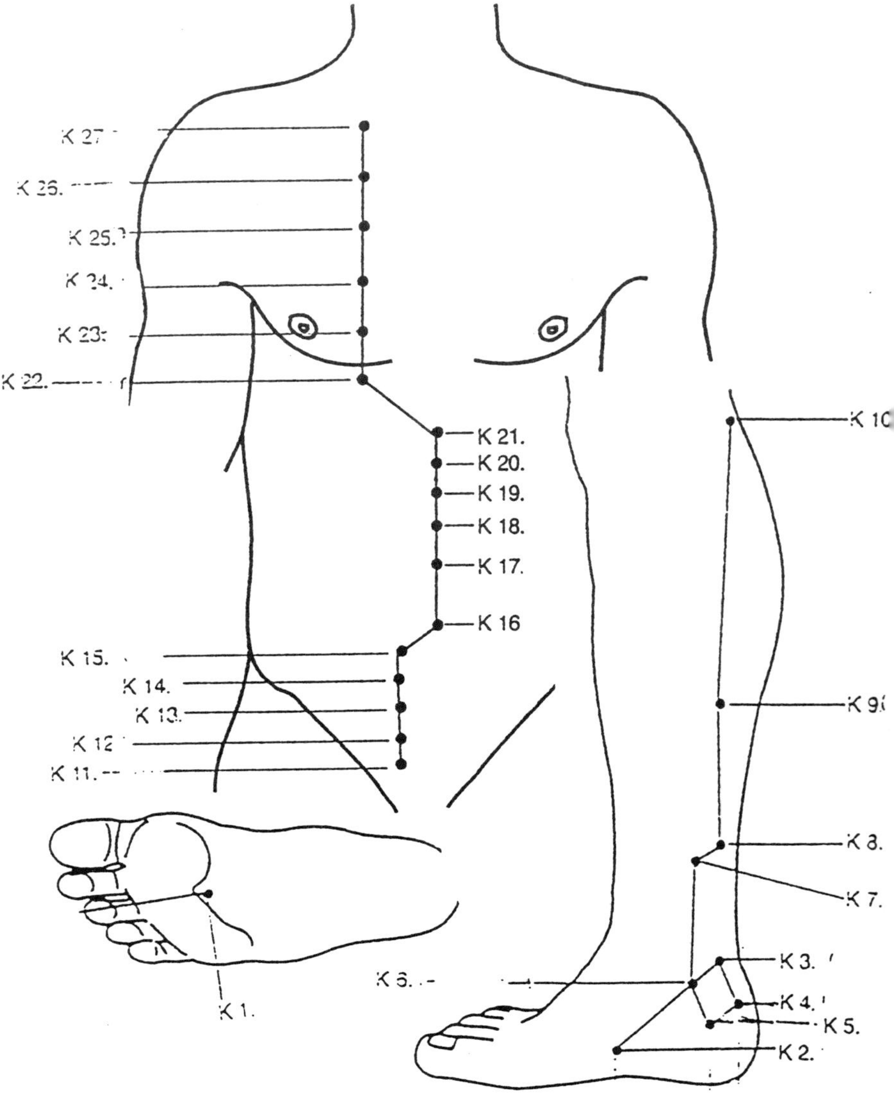

8. KIDNEY 足少陰腎經 K - (==) Lesser Yin

1. 용천 湧泉 •
2. 연곡 然谷 •
3. 태계 太谿 •
4. 대종 大鍾
5. 수천 水泉
6. 조해 照海 •
7. 부류 復溜 •
8. 교신 交信
9. 축빈 築賓
10. 음곡 陰谷 •
11. 횡골 橫骨
12. 대혁 大赫
13. 기혈 氣穴 •
14. 사만 四滿 •
15. 중주 中注 •
16. 황수 肓兪
17. 상곡 商曲
18. 석관 石關 •
19. 음도 陰都 •
20. 통곡 通谷 •
21. 유문 幽門
22. 보랑 步廊
23. 신봉 神封
24. 영허 靈墟
25. 신장 神藏
26. 욱중 彧中
27. 수부 兪府

9. CIRCULATION-SEX

P - (☰☰) Absolute Yin

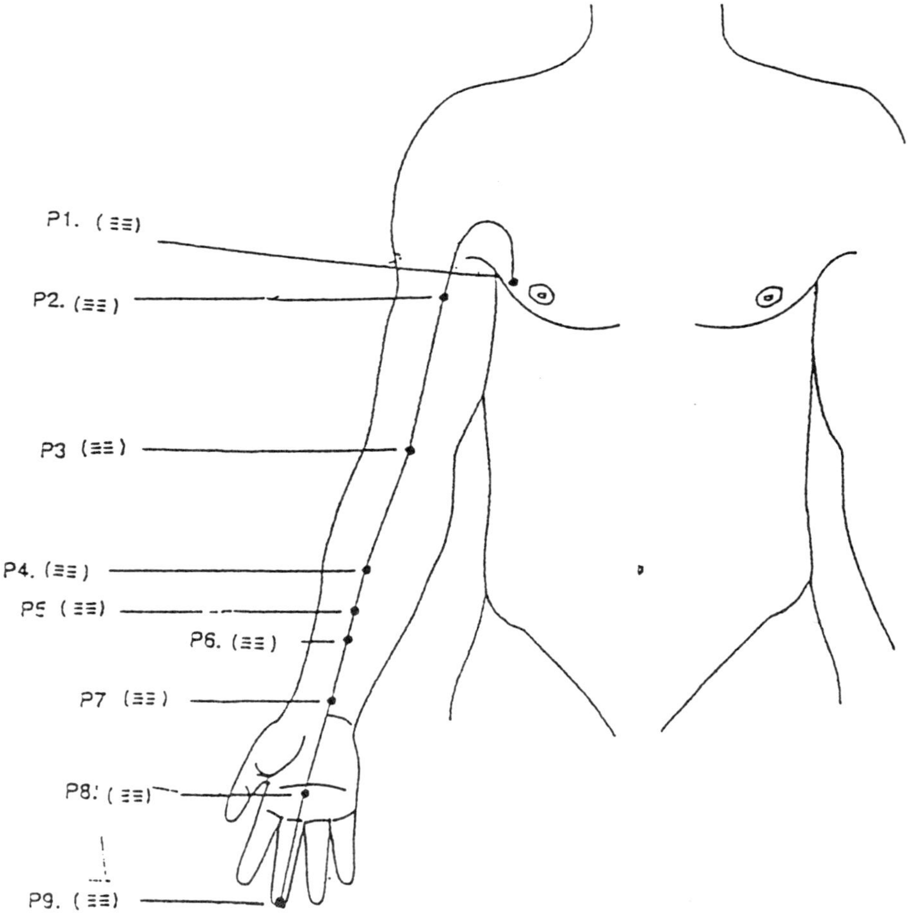

. Circulation-Sex 手厥陰心包經 P-(三)Aesolute Yin

1. 천지 天池

2. 천천 天泉

3. 곡택 曲澤 •

4. 극문 郄門

5. 간사 間使 •

6. 내관 內關 •

7. 대릉 大陵 •

8. 노궁 勞宮 •

9. 중충 中衝 •

10. TRIPLE WARMER T - (☵), Lesser Yang

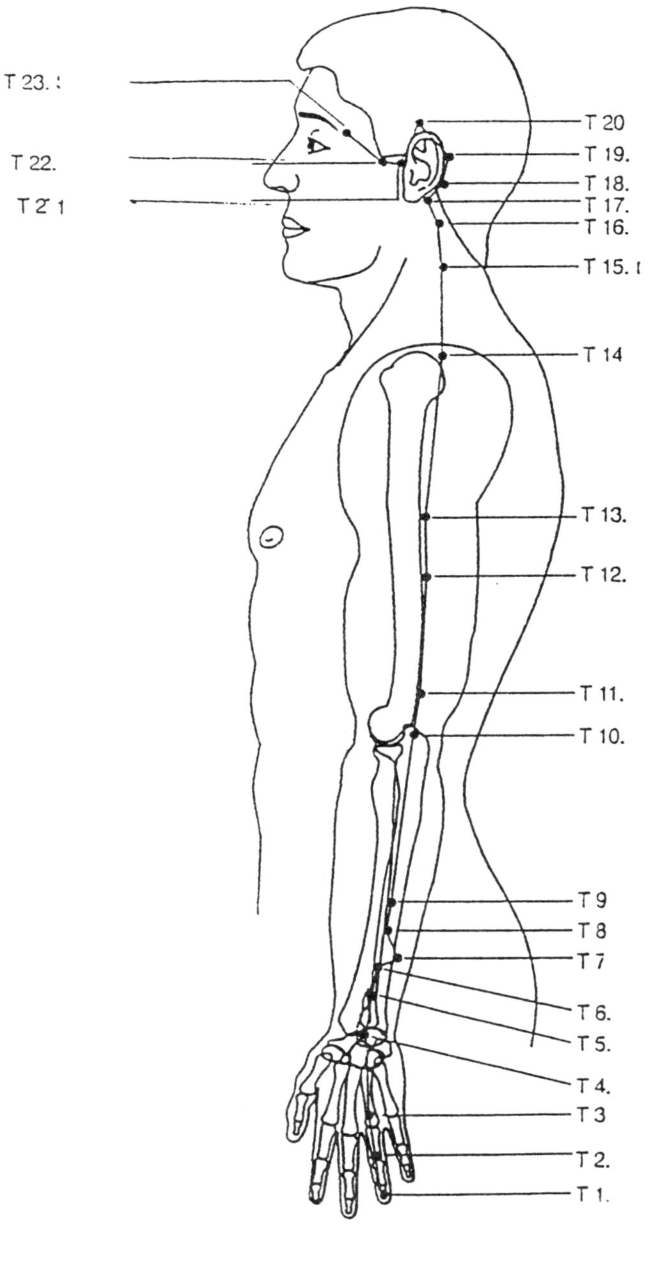

10. Triple Warmer 手少陽三焦經 T-( ) Lesser Yang

1. 관 충 關 衝 •
2. 액 문 液 門 •
3. 중 저 中 渚 •
4. 양 지 陽 池 •
5. 외 관 外 關 •
6. 지 구 支 溝 •
7. 회 종 會 宗
8. 삼양락 三陽絡
9. 사 독 四 瀆
10. 천 정 天 井 •
11. 청냉연 淸冷淵
12. 소 락 消 濼
13. 노 회 臑會
14. 견 료 肩 髎
15. 천 료 天 髎
16. 천 유 天 牖
17. 예 풍 翳 風 •
18. 계 맥 瘈 脈
19. 노 식 顱 息
20. 각 손 角孫
21. 이 문 耳門 •
22. 화 료 和 髎
23. 사죽공 絲竹空 •

11. GALL BLADDER

GB - (☱) Lesser Yang

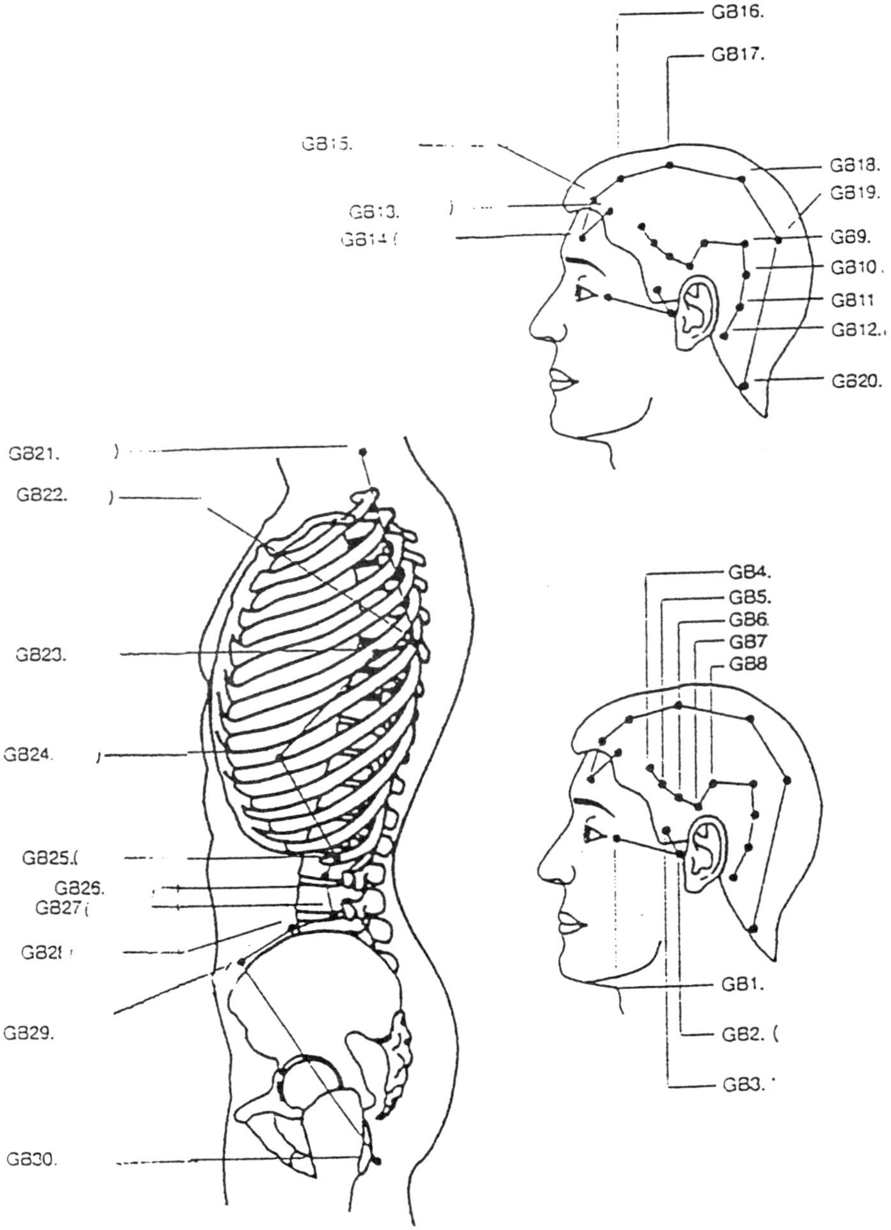

11. Gall Bladder 足少陽膽經 GB -(二) Lessor Yang

1. 동자료	瞳子髎	23. 첩 근	輒 筋
2. 청 회	聽 會 •	24. 일 월	日 月
3. 상 관	上 關	25. 경 문	京 門 •
4. 함 염	頷 厭 •	26. 대 맥	帶 脈 •
5. 현 로	懸 顱	27. 오 추	五 樞 •
6. 현 리	懸 釐	28. 유 도	維 道
7. 곡 빈	曲 鬢	29. 거 료	居 髎
8. 솔 곡	率 谷	30. 환 조	環 跳 •
9. 천 충	天 衝 •	31. 풍 시	風 市 •
10. 부 백	浮 白	32. 중 독	中 瀆 •
11. 규 음	竅 陰	33. 양 관	陽 關
12. 완 골	完 骨	34. 양능천	陽陵泉 •
13. 본 신	本 神 •	35. 양 교	陽 交 •
14. 양 백	陽 白 •	36. 외 구	外 丘
15. 임 읍	臨 泣	37. 광 명	光 明
16. 목 창	目 窓	38. 양 보	陽 輔
17. 정 영	正 營	39. 현 종	懸 鍾 •
18. 승 영	承 靈	40. 구 허	丘 墟 •
19. 뇌 공	腦 空	41. 임 읍	臨足泣 •
20. 풍 지	風 池 •	42. 지오회	地五會
21. 견 정	肩 井 •	43. 협 계	俠 谿 •
22. 연 액	淵 腋	44. 구 음	竅 陰 •

12. LIVER

LV - (☳) Absolute Yin

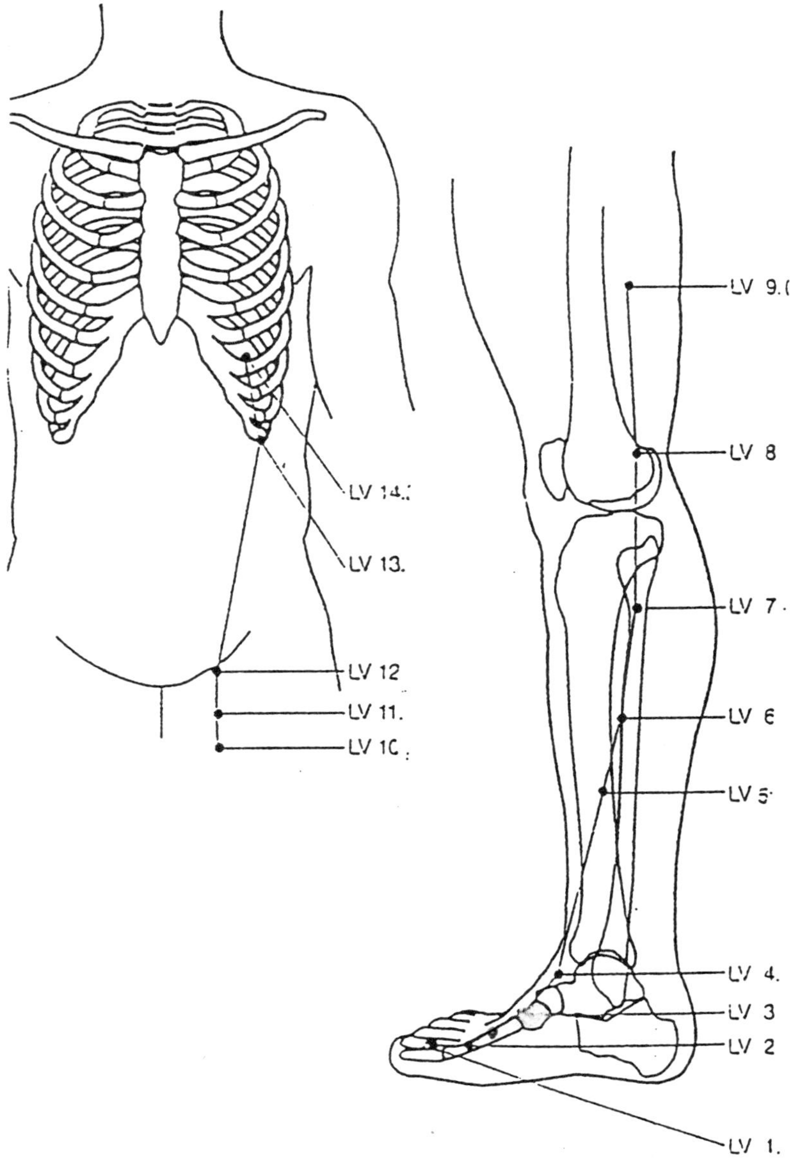

12. Liver 足厥陰肝經 LV-(三三) Absolute Yin

1.	대 돈	大 敦 •
2.	행 간	行間 •
3.	태 충	太衝 •
4.	중 봉	中 封 •
5.	여 구	蠡溝 •
6.	중 도	中 都 •
7.	슬 관	膝 關 •
8.	곡 천	曲 泉 •
9.	음 포	陰 包
10.	오 리	五 里
11.	음 렴	陰 廉
12.	급 맥	急 脈
13.	장 문	章 門 •
14.	기 문	期 門 •

13. GOVERNING VESSEL 督 脈 GV - (二) Greater Yang

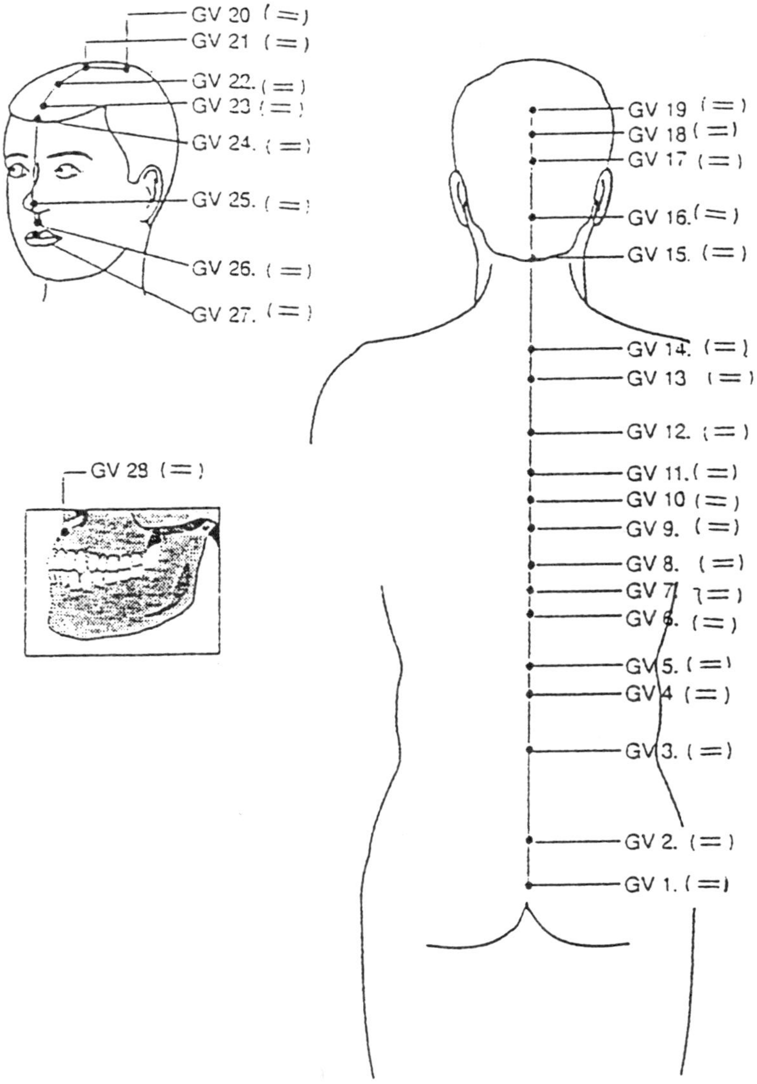

3. Governing Vessel 督脈. GV-(=) Greater Yang

1. 장 강	長强	•	15. 아 문	瘂門	•
2. 요 유	腰兪	•	16. 풍 부	風府	•
3. 양 관	陽關		17. 뇌 호	腦戶	
4. 명 문	命門	•	18. 강 간	强間	
5. 현 추	懸樞		19. 후 정	後頂	•
6. 척 중	脊中	•	20. 백 회	百會	•
7. 중 추	中樞		21. 전 정	前頂	•
8. 근 축	筋縮		22. 신 회	顖會	
9. 지 양	至陽		23. 상 성	上星	
10. 영 대	靈台		24. 신 정	神頂	•
11. 신 도	身道		25. 소 요	素髎	
12. 신 주	身柱	•	26. 수 구	水溝	•
13. 도 도	陶道	•	27. 태 단	兌端	
14. 대 추	大椎	•	28. 은 교	齦交	

14. CONCEPTION VESSEL   CV - (==) Greater Yin

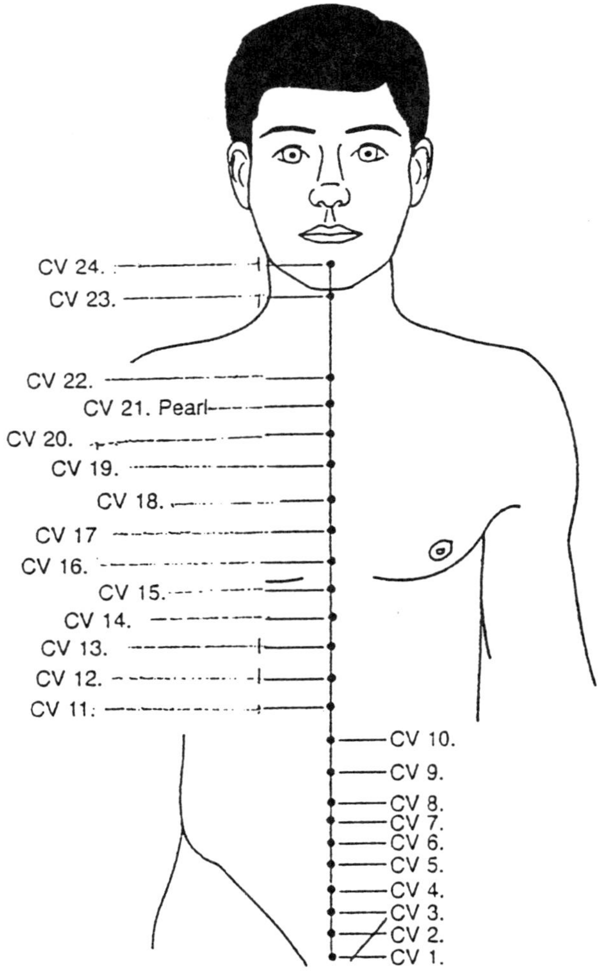

14. C0nception Vessel 任 脈 CV-(==)Greater Yin

1. 회음 會陰
2. 곡골 曲骨
3. 중극 中極 •
4. 관원 關元 •
5. 석문 石門 •
6. 기해 氣海 •
7. 음교 陰交 •
8. 신궐 神闕 •
9. 수분 水分
10. 하완 下脘 •
11. 건리 建里 •
12. 중완 中脘 •
13. 상완 上脘 •
14. 거궐 巨闕 •
15. 구미 鳩尾
16. 중정 中庭
17. 전중 膻中
18. 옥당 玉堂
19. 자궁 紫宮
20. 화개 華蓋
21. 선기 璇璣
22. 천돌 天突 •
23. 염천 廉泉
24. 승장 承漿 •

1. LUNGS 手太陰肺經 L - (二二) Greater Yin

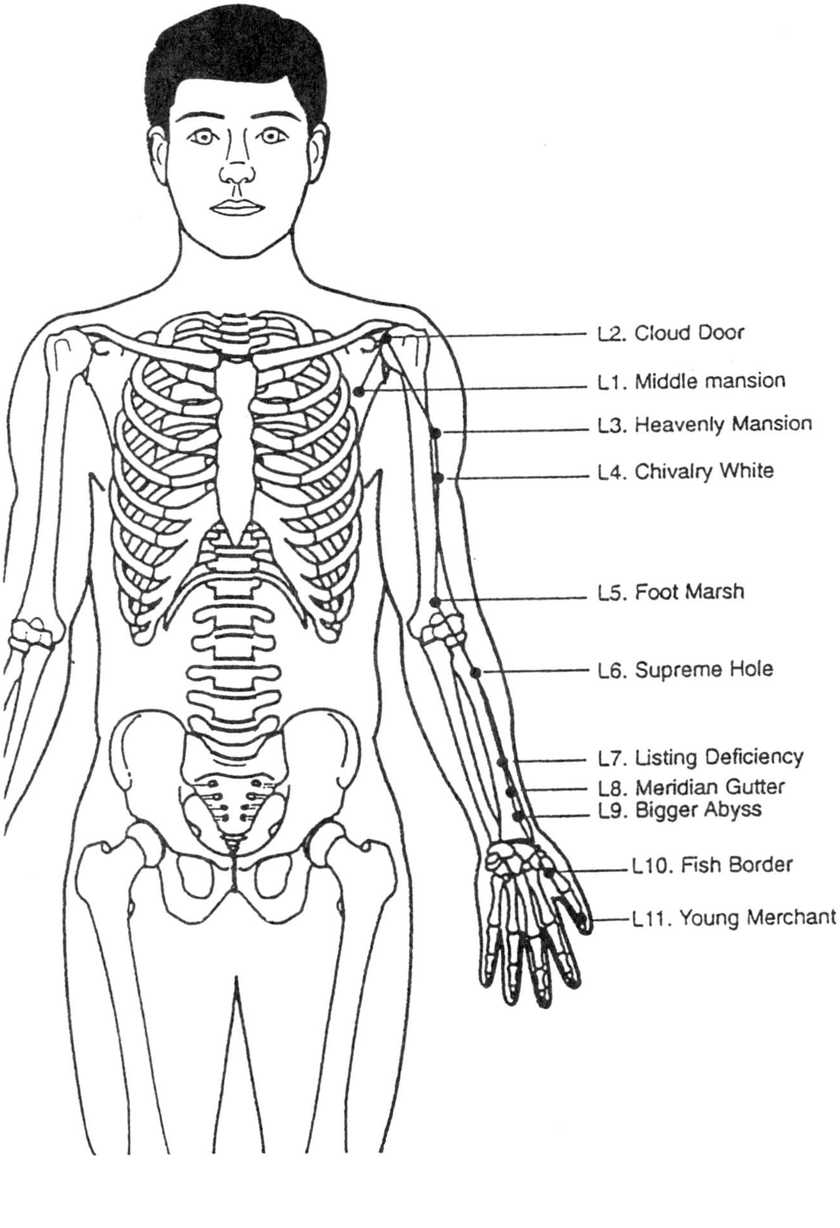

2. LARGE INTESTINE 手陽明大腸經 LI - (☰) Sun-Light Yang

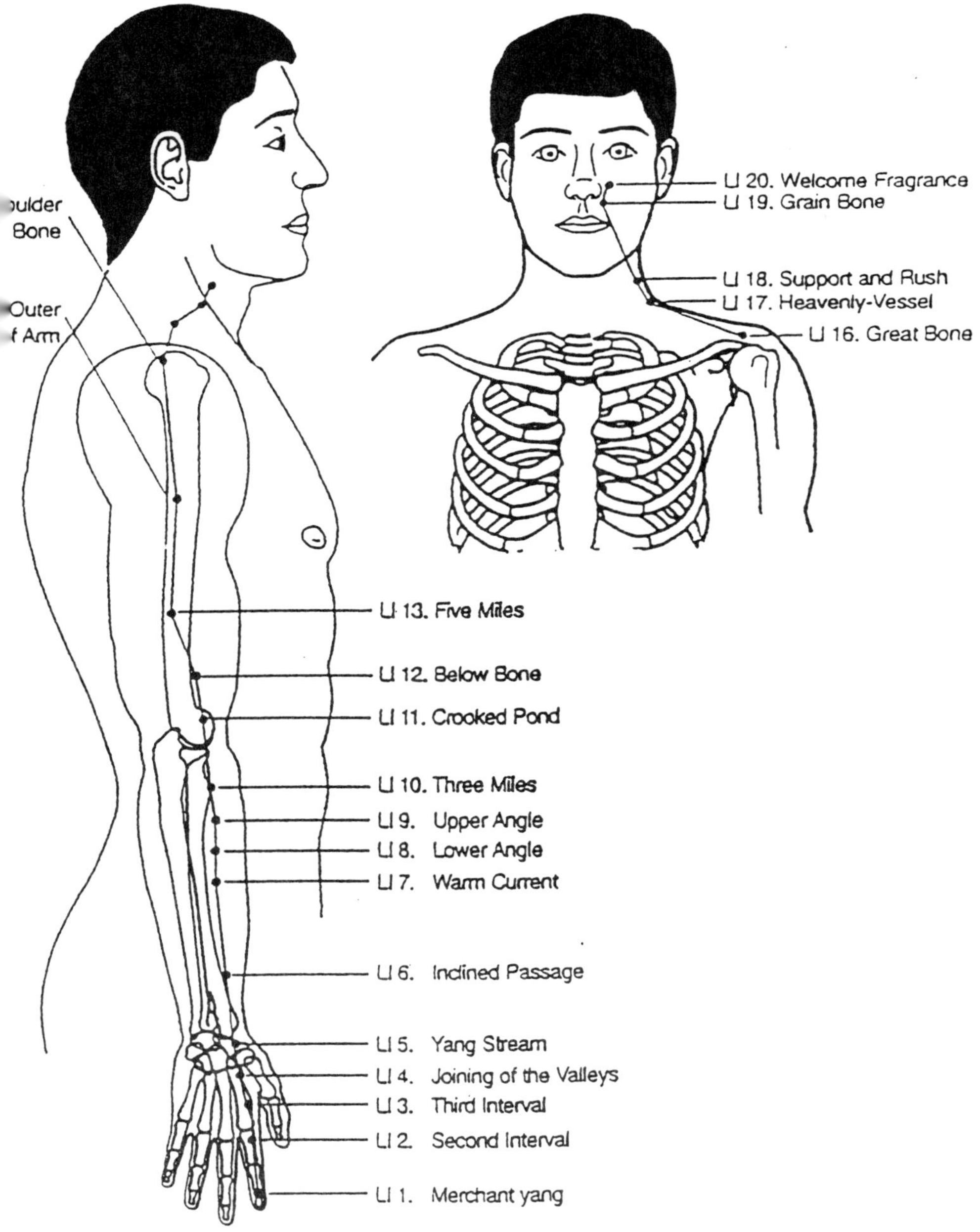

3. STOMACK 足陽明胃經 S - (三) Sun-Light Yang

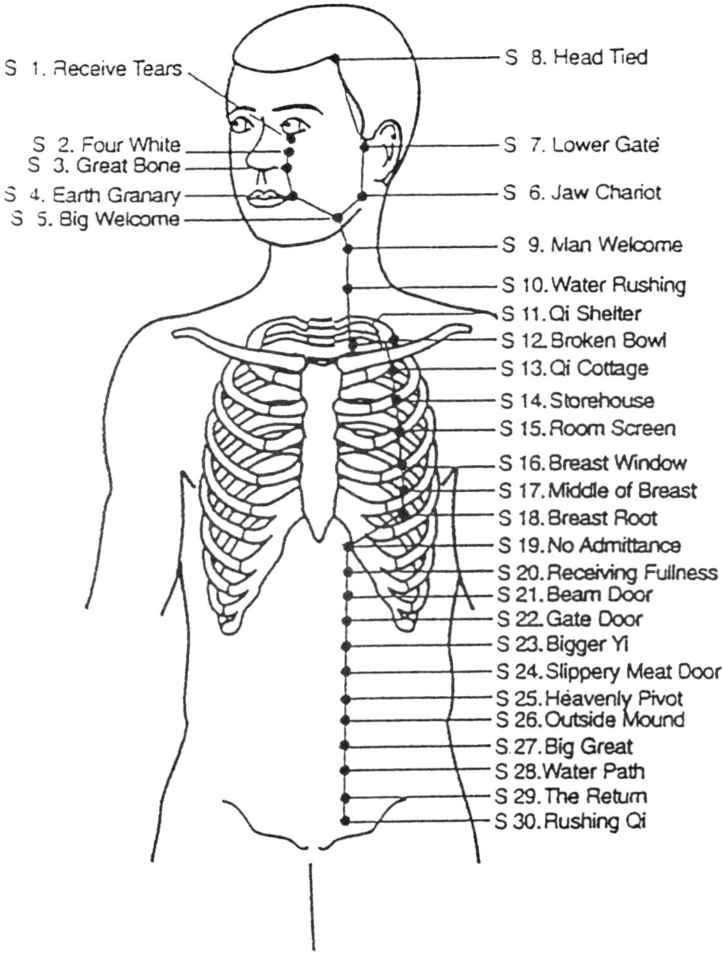

3. STOMACK 足陽明胃經 S - (☰) Sun-Light Yang B

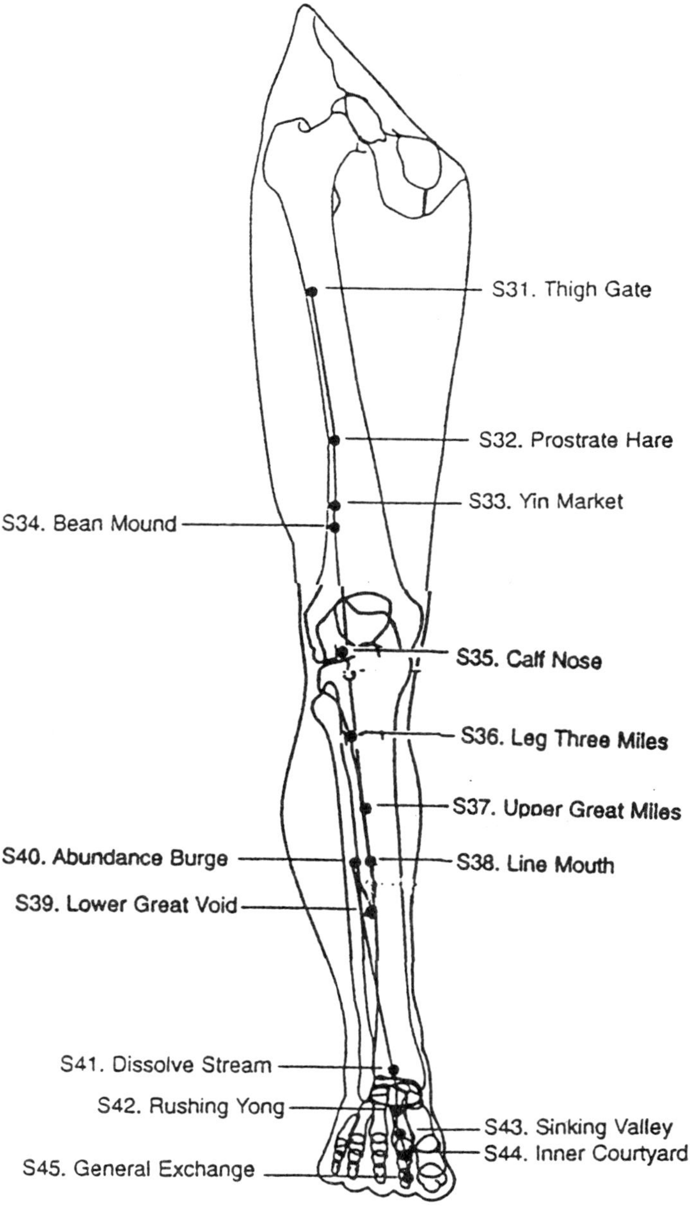

4. SPLEEN 足太陰脾經 SP - (==) Greater Yin

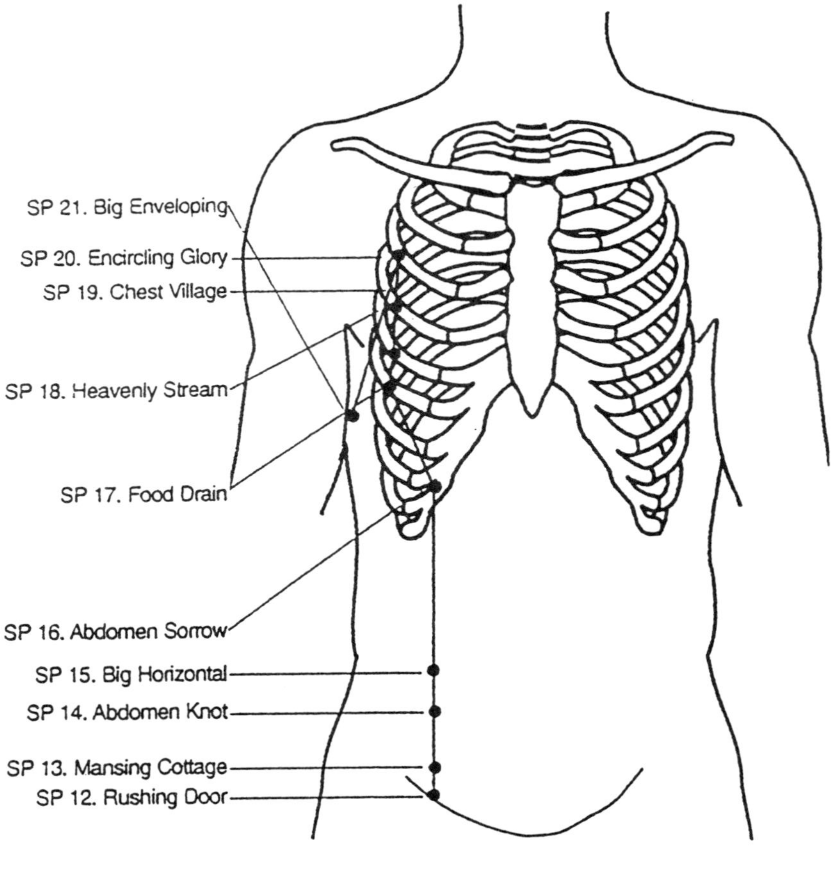

4. SPLEEN 足太陰脾經 SP - (==) Greater Yin B

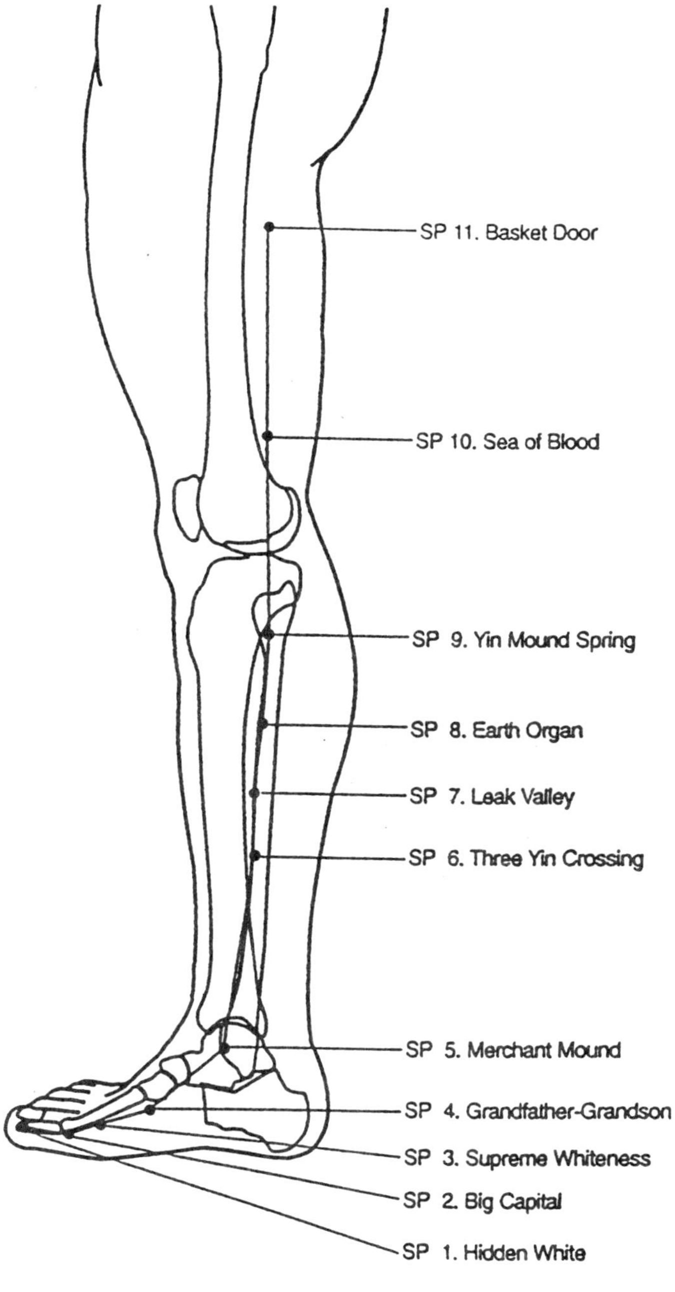

5. HEART 手少陰心經 H - (⚍) Lesser Yin

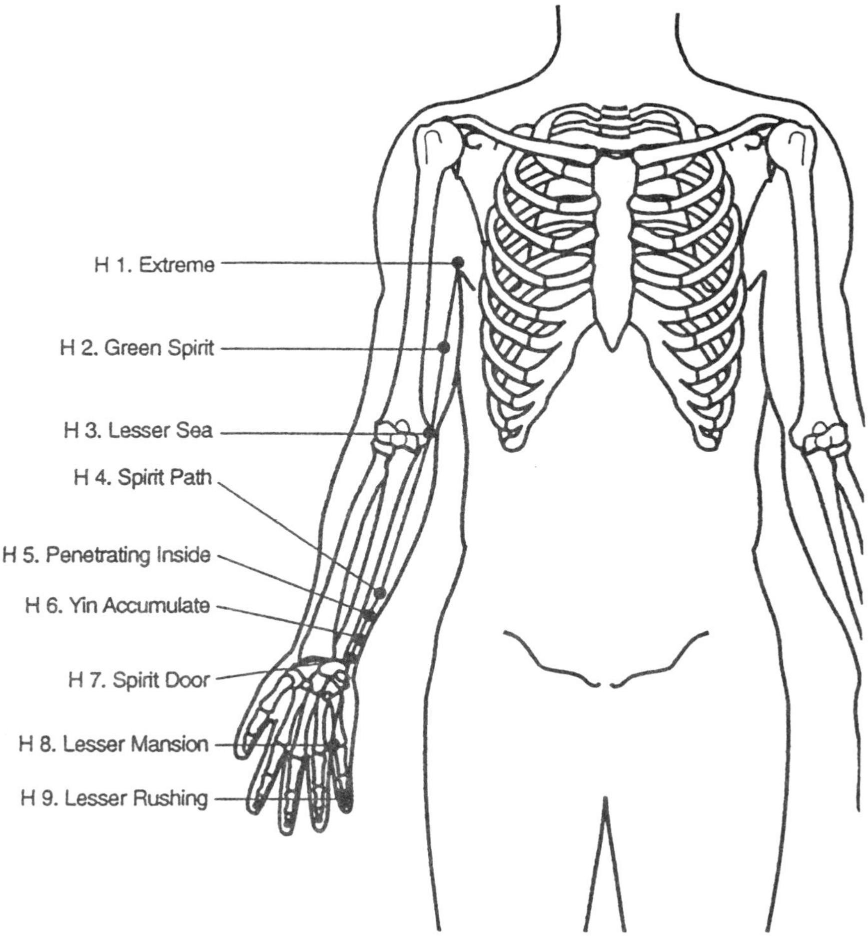

6. SMALL INTESTINE 手太陽小腸經 SI - (═) GREATER Yang

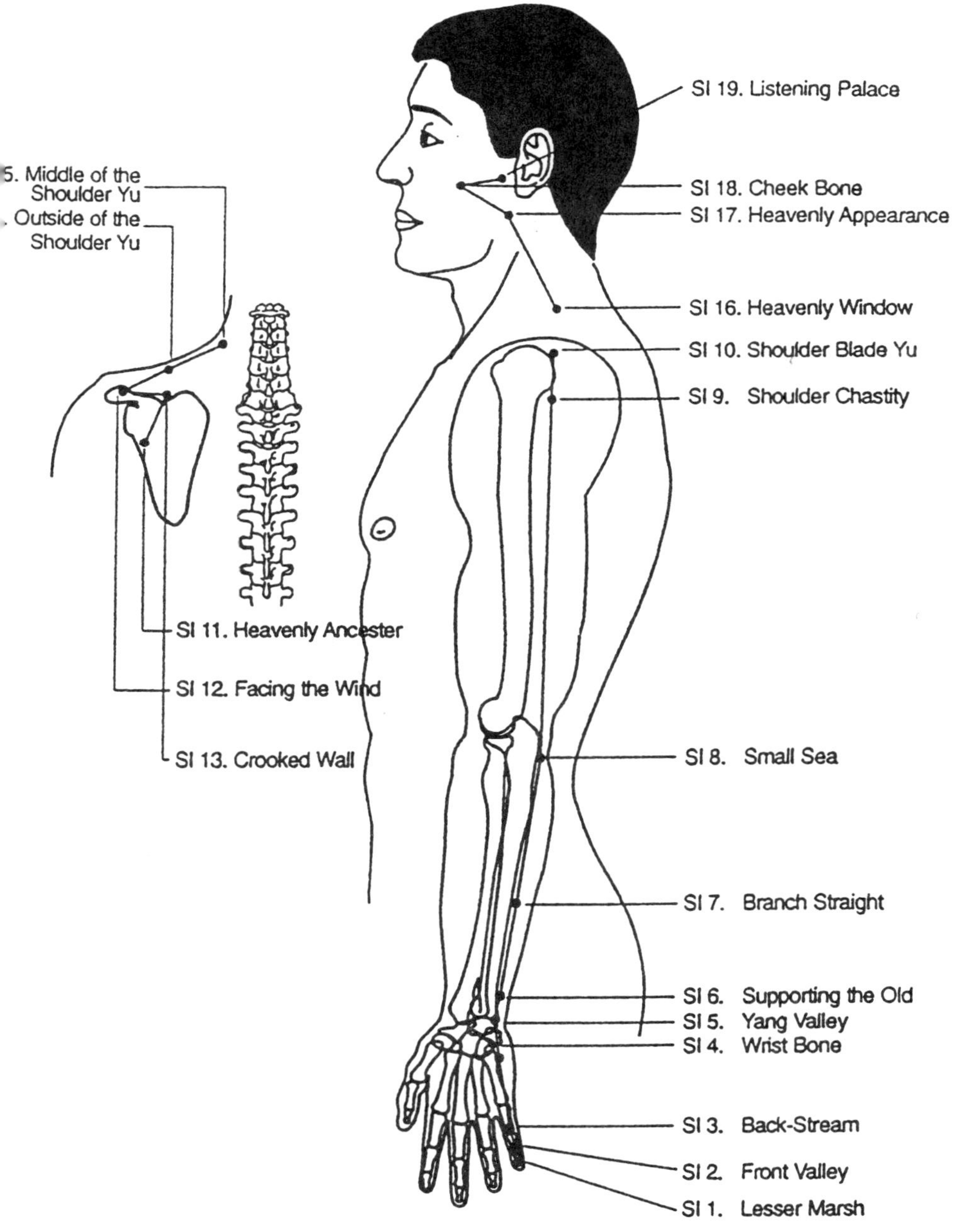

7. BLADDER 足太陽膀胱經 B - (=) Greater Yang A

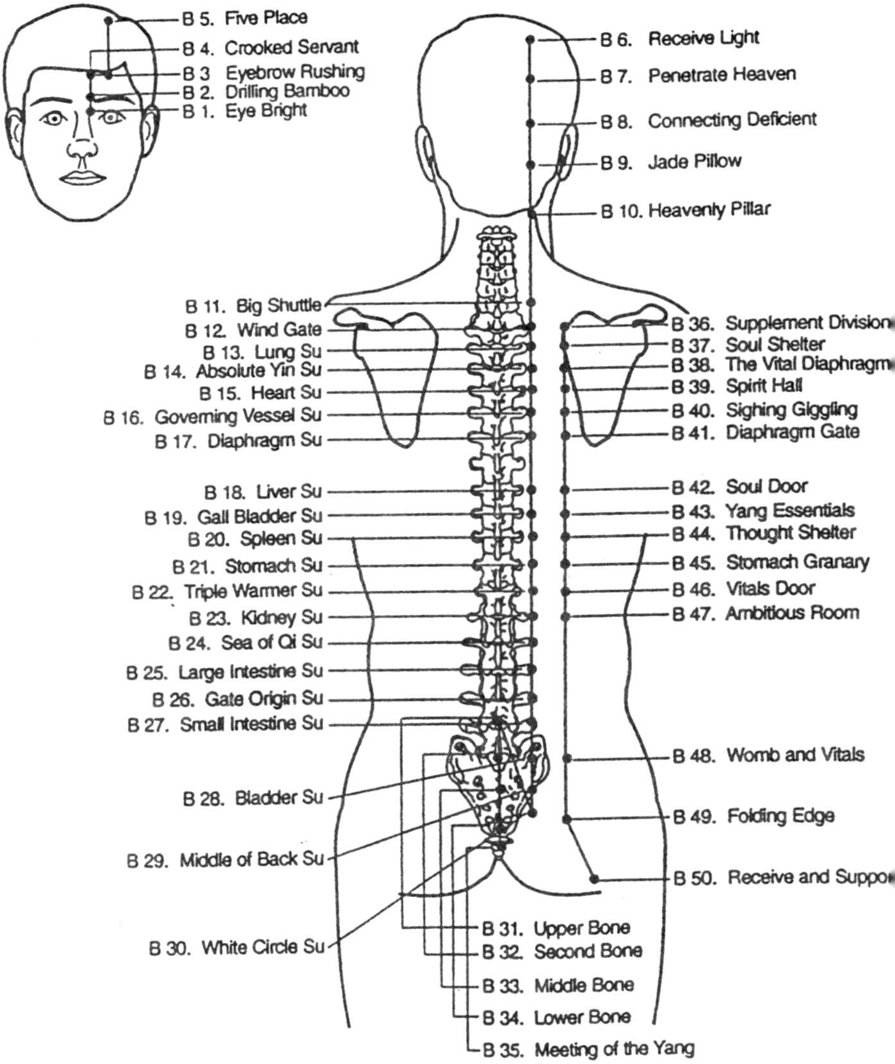

7. BLADDER 足太陽膀胱經 B - (三) Greater Yang

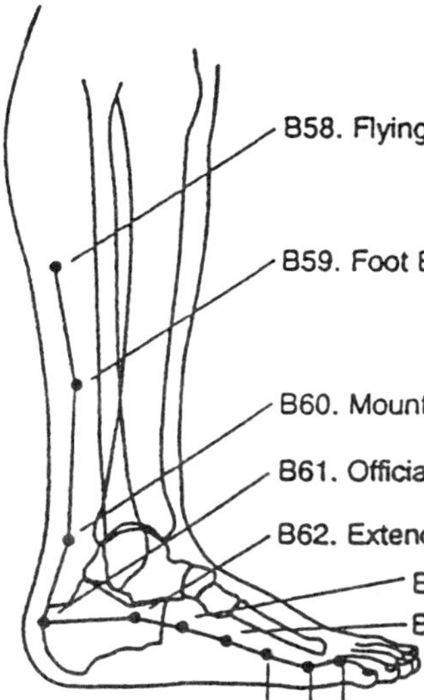

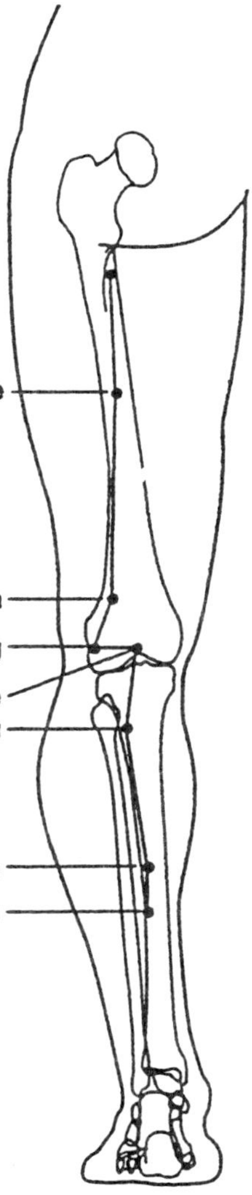

8. KIDNEY 足少陰腎經 K - (==) Lesser Yin A

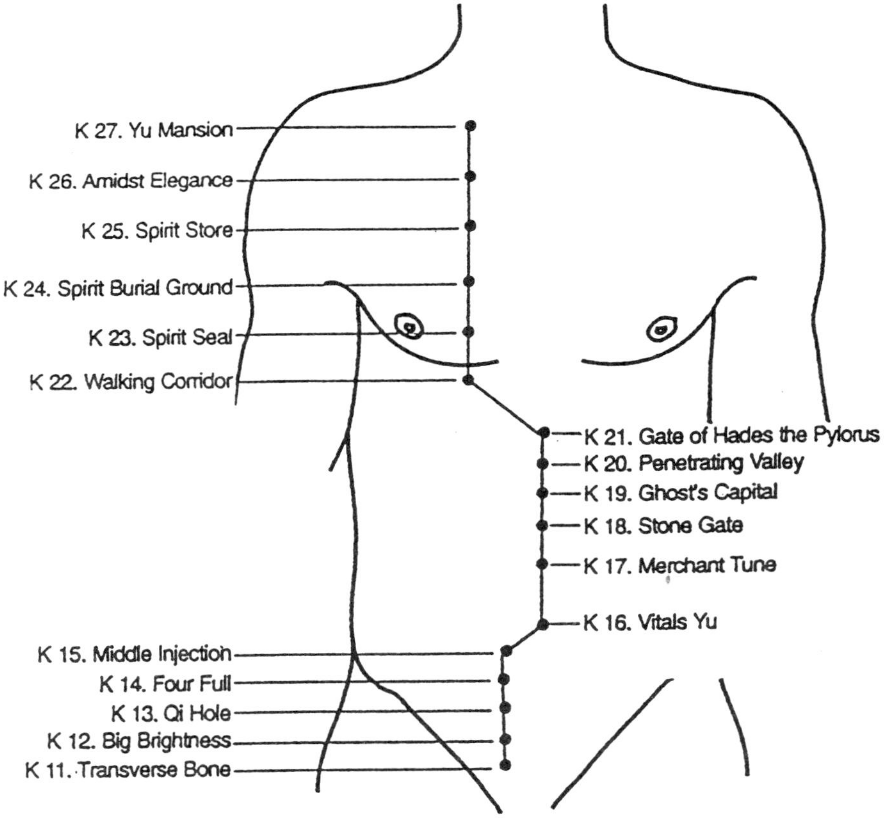

8. KIDNEY 足少陰腎經 K - (==) Lesser Yin B

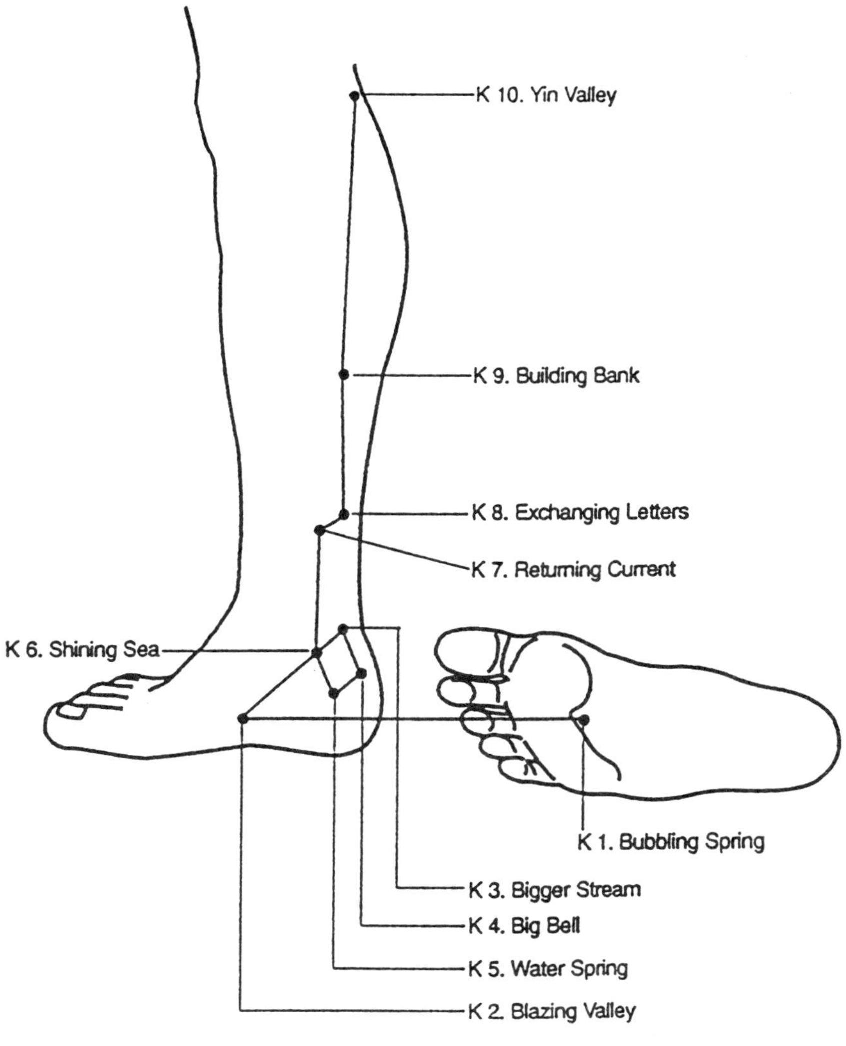

9. CIRCULATION-SEX 手厥陰心包經 P - (☰☰) Absolute Yin

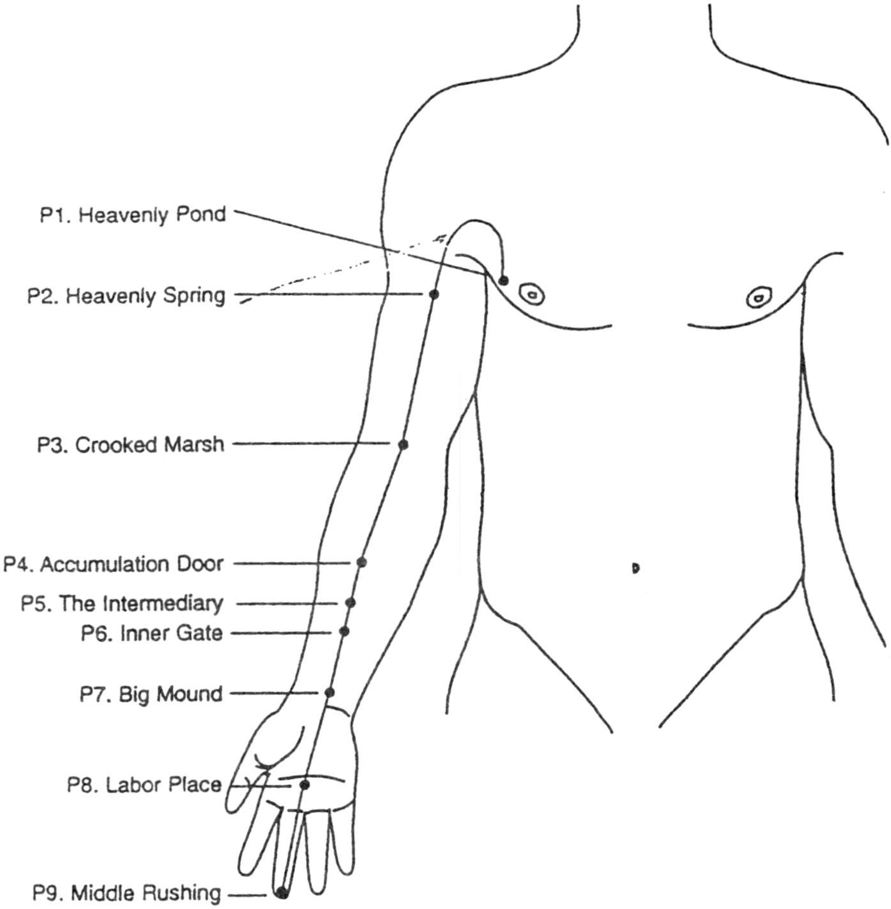

10. TRIPLE WARMER 手少陽三焦經 T - (⚏) Lesser Yang

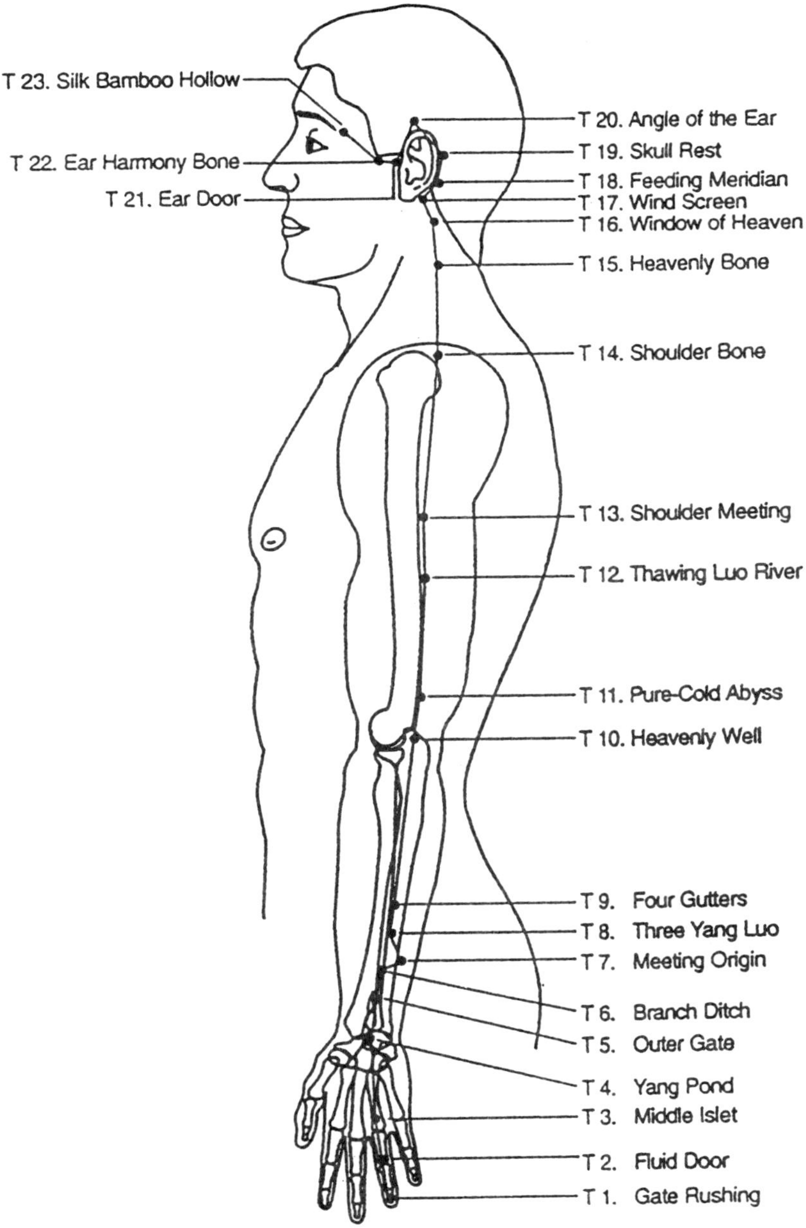

11. GALL BLADDER 足少陽胆經 GB - (☴) Lesser Yang

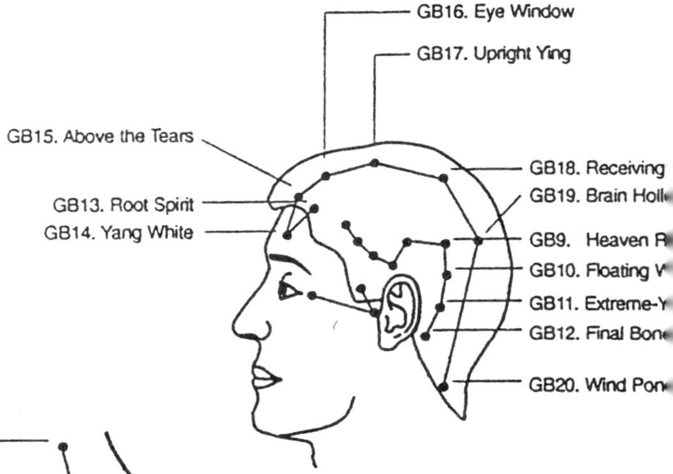

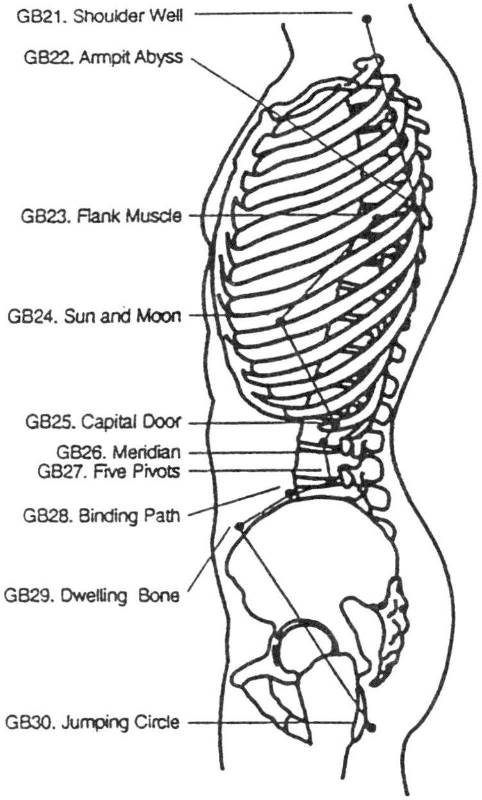

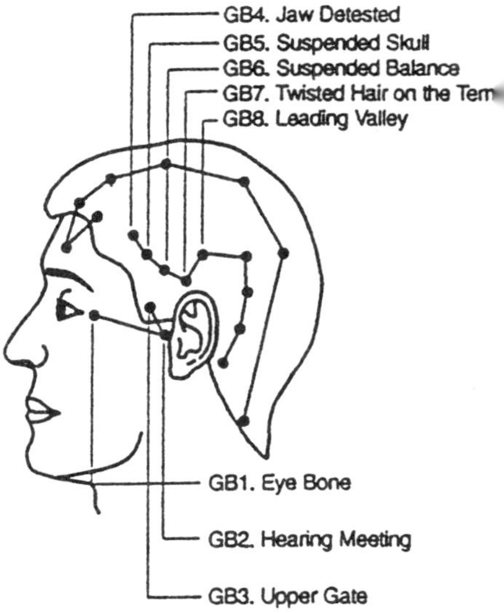

11. GALL BLADDER 足少陽胆經 GB - (==) Lesser Yang B

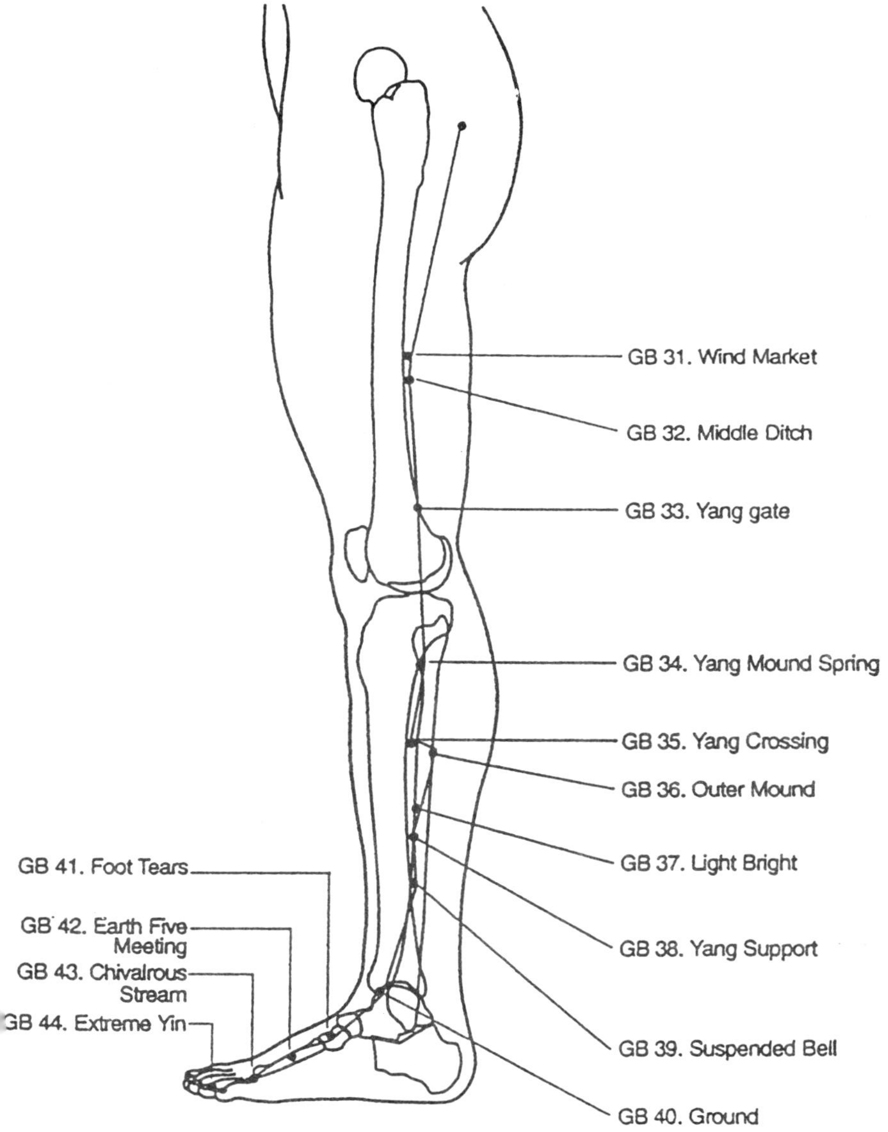

12. LIVER 足厥陰肝經 LV - (☳) Absolute Yin

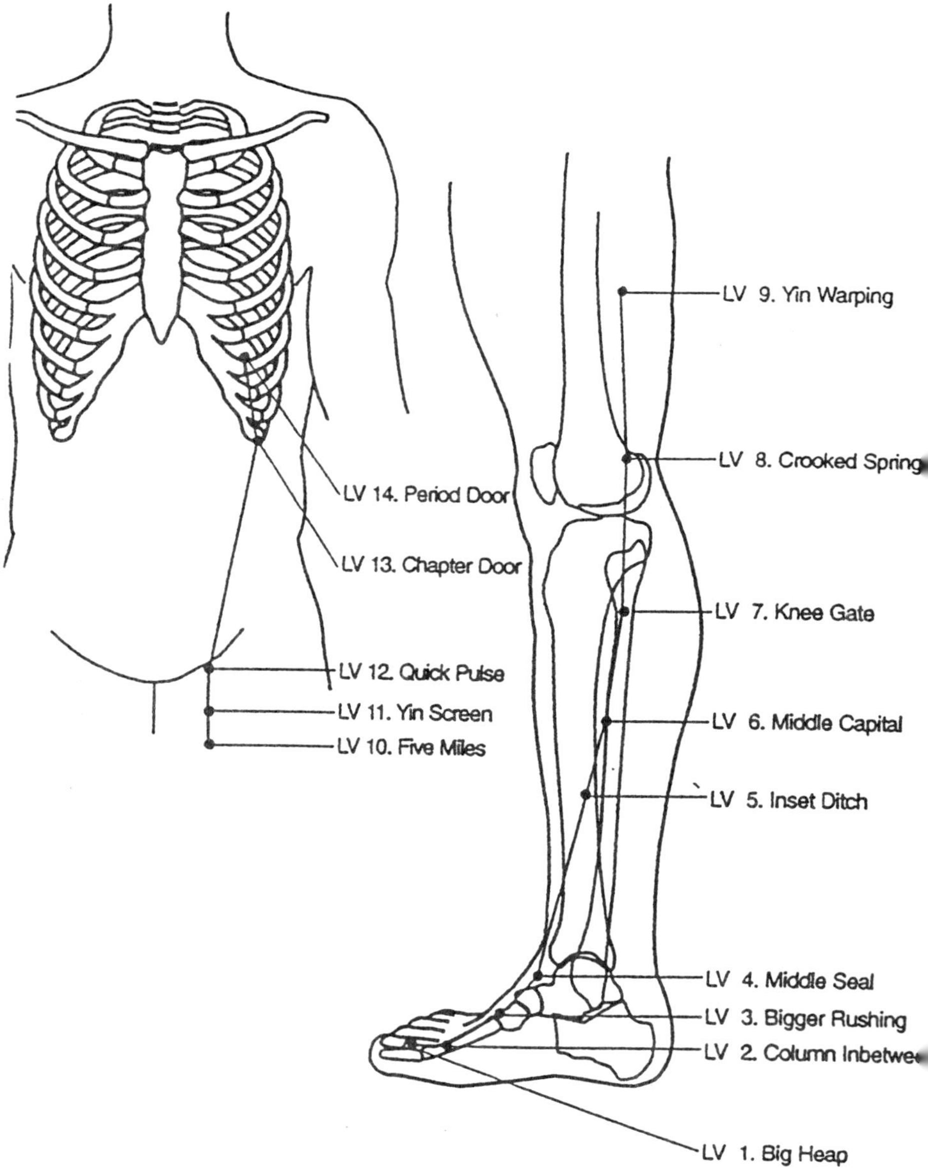

3. GOVERNING VESSEL 督脈 GV - (═) Greater Yang

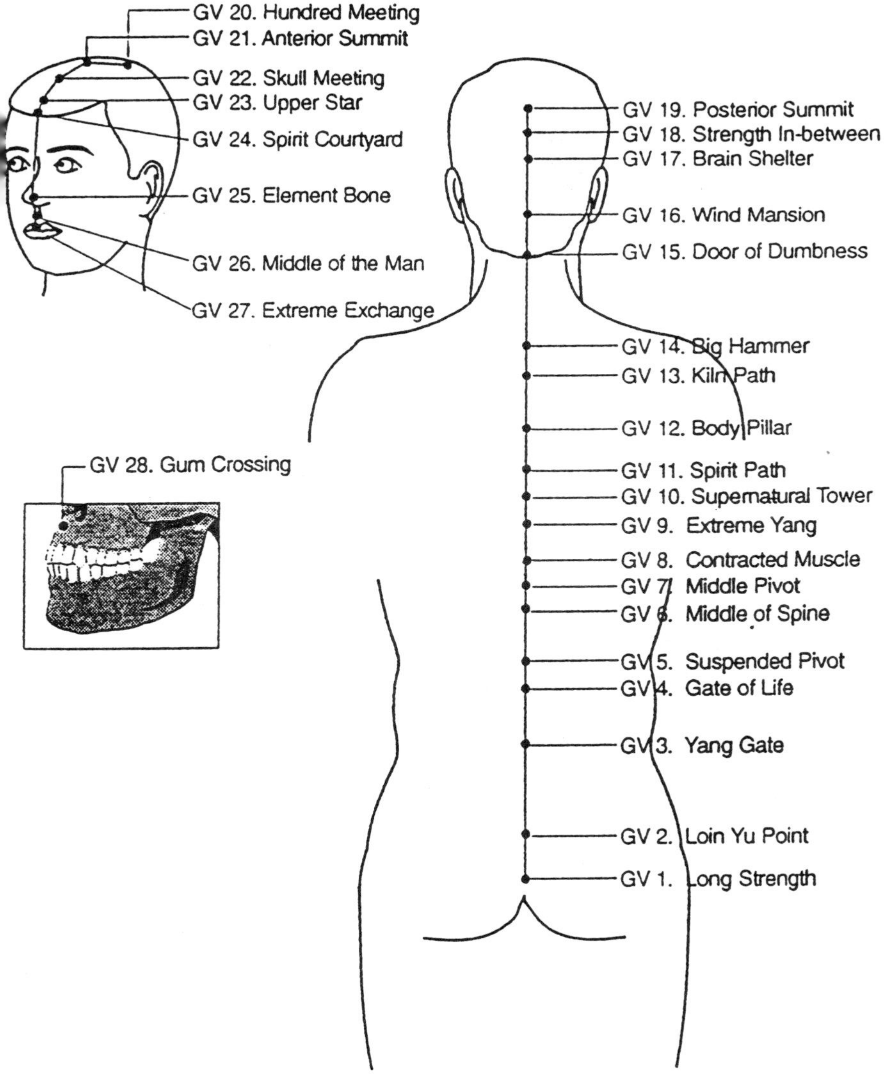

14. CONCEPTION VESSEL 任 脈 CV - (☷) Greater Yin

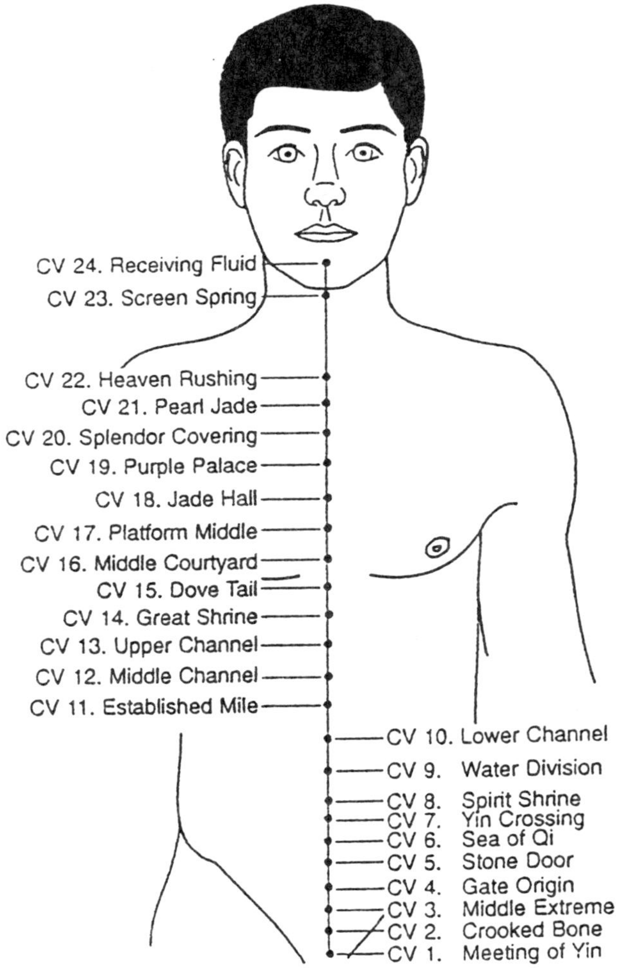

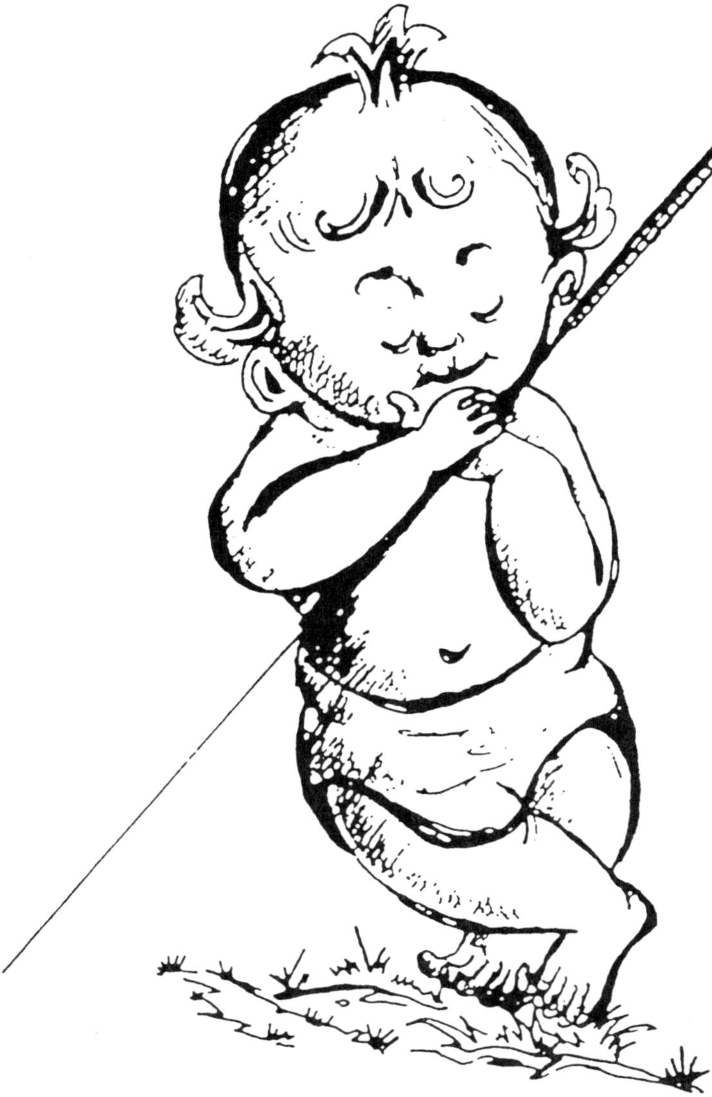

(Reference:from the book by Yoshio, Nagahama)

METHODS OF APPLYING ACUPUNCTURAL NEEDLES

1. TYPES AND CHARACTERISTICS OF ACUPUNCTURAL NEEDLES

(1) Nine Types of Needles:

In the Yung-Goo Volume One, the oldest medical book from ancient China, nine types of Acupunctural needles are distinguished. Of these nine, Bong-chim and Pah-chim were later designated as Sam-Nung-chims, which were used as a kind of surgical tools to open protuberant spots and to relieve the congested blood in certain parts of human body.

Today, the most widely employed needle is Ho-chim, which is, however, not used to relieve the blood congestion. Other types of needles, such as Wonchim(round needle) and Shik-chim, are employed to apply special stimulation(pressure) to the skin-surface, but not used for insertion. Even today, some practitioners still employ these needles in their original usage, but these needles may be viewed as an modified version of So-ah-chim (infant-needle or skin-needle), which is commonly employed today.

(2) Sam-Nung-Chim(three-sided needle):

The needle-shaft is of round-shaped, but the needle-point is three-sided. The length of the needle is about one and one half inches. It is usually made of stainless steel. It is generally used to relieve the blood-congestion, but the one with dull point can be used as a skin-needle.

(3) Ho-Chim:

This is currently popular in use. To the one half inch long shaft is attached a slender metallic needle with a sharp point.
The length of the needle-body is between five twelveths of an inch to three inches, but one to two inches (3-6 centimeters) in length are quite common. The length of needle employed depends upon the purpose and the user's preference, but it is customary to employ the one with the length of one and one quarter inches to one and one half. The diameters of the needles are numbered from one to ten, as shown below:

Number	Diameter i millimeters (one millimeter = .03937 inch)
#1 needle	about 0.170
#2 needle	about 0.185
#3 needle	about 0.200
#4 needle	about 0.220
#5 needle	about 0.235
#6 needle	about 0.260
#7 needle	about 0.280
#8 needle	about 0.300
#9 needle	about 0.310
#10 needle	about 0.320

Of these numbered needles, the numbers 3,4,and 5 are the most commonly used.

These needles are much thinner when compared with the thinnest hypodermic needle--0.41 millimeter in diameter. If a moderate stimulation is required for any Acupunctural treatment, it is preferable to employ a thin needle. There are also many different qualities of Acupunctural needles: gold-needles, silver-needles, San-Boo-Rah needles, stainless-steel needles, etc. Of these, the silver-needles are widely employed. For the purpose of providing a mild stimulation, the gold-needle is commonly used, whereas for stronger stimulation steel-needle or San-Boo-Rah needle is used.
The needle-point can be called the life of Ho-chim, and its effectiveness greatly affects the Acupunctural insertion.

II. METHODS OF APPLYING ACUPUNCTURAL NEEDLES

There are three ways of applying Ho-chim needles: The traditional Chinese way of twisting method, the tapping method, and tube-needle method. The tapping method involves the tapping of needles by a tiny hammer, but it is seldom used today. The commonly used methods today are the twisting and the tube needle.

(1) Yeun-chim Method(twisting needle):

First, use the thumb and index-finger of the right-hand to hold the needle-shaft. Second, put the thumb-tip of the left hand on the treatment-point and place the needle-point lightly touching the skin surface while the needle-body is leaning against the thumb-ball of the left hand and the index finger's tip of the right hand is steadying the needle in place. Third, press the needle into the skin of the treatment-point by the right hand, while simultaneously put the pressure on the left hand's thumb in the same direction of the needle. This procedure is called "skin penetration" or tan-ip. It is better to administer skin penetration in one motion. The left hand steadily holding the needle is called "pressing hand", whereas the right hand is termed "inserting hand". The "pressing hand" plays the role of minimizing the pain at the moment of needle insertion.

The "inserting hand" is to twist the inserted needle sideway, while "the pressing hand" is to provide the pressure until the needle-point being inserted into the proper depth. At the prescribed depth some appropriate stimulation must be given before extracting the needle by the right hand. Once becoming familiarized with the procedures, the Acupuncturist presses the skin surface with the pressing hand, while the needle is inserted by pressing the needle shaft with the inserting hand. Some practitioners dip the needle point into mercury before insertion in order to have a smooth penetration.

(2) Tube Needle Method:

Put the needle into the needle tube and hold it steady by the right hand in such a way that the needle point does not stick out from the tube, while the pressing fingers of the left hand hold the tip of the tube and place it right on the skin of the Acupunctural point. Then, use the index finger's tip of the right hand to tap mildly once or twice the head of the needle shaft. In other words, the skin is punctured when the head of needle shaft disappears into the needle tube. Subsequently, the tube is taken out while the left hand is holding the needle point, and then ,the needle insertion is made with the right hand by applying the twisting method. There are two methods of putting the needle into the tube: two hand method and one hand method.

Two Hand Method: This method involves the putting the needle shaft's end into the tube while the right hand is holding the tube and the left hand is holding the needle. It is a very simple procedure so that practice is not necessary to master the method. However, this method has the disadvantage of time consuming, when many needles are to be inserted around the treatment point.

One hand Method: This method involves the procedure of holding the needle tube in-between the small and the middle finger and of using the thumb and index finger to pull the needle shaft into the tube. This method requires some practice. Once the procedure is mastered, it can be repeated 25 to 30 times in a minute.

III. THE SKILLS OF NEEDLE INSERTION

There are many different technique of needle

insertion. The resonance of needle stimulation (very important) may be strong or mild depending upon the skillful hand manipulation of Acupunctural needles.

(1)Simple Straight Insertion:

This is the most elementary of Acupunctural methods. The needle is pressed into the treatment point without twisting manipulation and then,extracted rather slowly. When the needle is inserted and extracted slowly, it causes a very mild resonant stimulation around the treatment point.
There are other traditional methods of insertion:Soo-chim-sool(inserting and extracting at the breathing interval);Awk-noo-sool(rapid insertion for five minutes);Sam-cho-sool(one minute insertion and repeat this tree times).

(2)Twisting Insertion:

The needle insertion and extraction are made by twisting the needle side way just like the winding of the wrist watch. This is called Suhn-yul-sool. Another method is to twist the needle to the right or the left at insertion, whereas at its extraction the needle is twisted in the opposite direction. This is called Hwae-suhn-sool. If twisted slowly, the resonance of the needle stimulation would be mild, whereas if twisted rapidly, the resonance would be more stronger.

(3)Pecking-Bird Method:

Having inserted the needle into the prescribed depth at the treatment point, this hand manipulation of needle involves the rapid insertion extraction of the needle resembling a bird's pecking motion. When, with the needle being kept inserted, the needle is twisted about as well as thrusted in all four directions, it is called Nam-chim-sool(wild insertion method).

Both methods are intended to arouse strong resonant stimulation.

(4)Needle-Being-Kept-Inserted Method:

When the needle point reaches the prescribed depth, it is kept there for twenty to thirty seconds in cases of short treatment, or twenty to thirty minutes in cases of long treatment. There are two techniques of needle manipulation:one way is to insert several needles around the treatment point and to push-pull them alternatively, the so called Kyo-ho-chi-chim, and the other way is to occasionally apply the Pecking Bird Method while the needle is being kept inserted, the so called Jack-do-chi-chim. The keeping of the inserted needle at the prescribed depth for some duration is to continuously provide mild resonant stimulation at the treatment point, which is intended to cure cold symptom due to poor blood circulation and to ease the state of excitement.

(5)Push-Pull Method:

This method involves the following procedure: Pulling up a little of the inserted needle and reinsert it to the prescribed depth. The are four varieties of this method.
Sam-bup-sool: Pull up a little of the inserted needle and reinsert it once to the fore and once to the aft.
Sah-pahng-chun-sool: Twisting the needle point to the right and left twice each at an angled front direction.
Sah-pahng-in-sool: Reinsert sideway four times.
Sah-pahng-ji-sool: Reinsert four times at an inclined direction.

All of these varieties would provide slightly stronger resonant stimulation at the treatment point.

(6) Wave-Like-Stimulation Method:

This method involves the stimulation of the inserted needle. It is to provide a mild wave-like stimulation. There are four varieties of this method.
Yul-haeng-sool: Use the nail of the thumb or of the index finger of the right hand to tap the needle shaft.
Neh-joe-sool: Tap the needle shaft by the needle tube.
Kee-paek-sool: Tap the side of the needle by the needle tube.
On-chim-sool: Put the pressure by the pressing-hand in all four directions(fore,aft,right,and left).

PRECAUTIONS ON ACUPUNCTURAL TREATMENT

1. Do not take any alcoholic beverages or any drinks containing stimulant when Acupunctural treatment is administered.

2. Do not give Acupunctural treatment before or after any medication (drugs) or hypodermic injection.

3. Do not give Acupunctural treatment when the patient is extremely hungry or had a full meal.

4. Avoid sexual intercourse before or after Acupunctural treatment.

5. Do not give Acupunctural treatment to the patients having legally defined contagious diseases.

6. Take a special precaution when Acupuncturaltreatment is to be administered to women with pregnancy of more than six months.

7. Bath or shower should not be taken with three hours of Acupunctural treatment.

-REFERENCE-

1. Ahn, Jong Woo, The Basic Acupuncture, 1970.

2. Chae, Fang, Methods of Acupuncture, 1969.

3. Chan, Pedro, Acupuncture: Electro-Acupuncture Anesthesisa, 1972.

4. Chinese Acupunctural Medical School, The Textbook of Acupuncture, 1971.

5. Chinese Medical Research Assoiation, The New Handbook on Acupunctural Points, 1972.

6. Choi, Yong Tae and Lee, Soo Ho, Precise of Acupunctural and Moxibustion, 1974.

7. Commercial Printing Company(Hong Kong), The Basic Knowledge of Acupuncture, 1970.

8. ______, The Handbook of Acupuncture, 1971.

9. ______, The Acupunctural Points for the Ear, 1972.

10. Creator Company, Encyclopedia of Chinese Acupuncture, 1972.

11. Duke, Mark, Acupuncture, 1972.

12. Foreign Languages Press, Acupuncture Anaesthesia, 1972.

13. ______, Exploring the Secrets of Treating Deaf-Mutes, 1972.

14. Hashimoto, M, Japanese Acupuncture, 1968.

15. Hoh,Joon,Traditional Medical Secrets from the East,1968.

16. Hohn Eem, History of Acupuncture,1970.

17. Honma Shyohaku,Gides to Acupunctural Treatment, 1944.

18. Horn, Joshua S.,Away With All Pests,1969.

19. Hyang, Pa Gusa,The Cardinal Principle of the Human Acupuncture.

20. Im,Ga Bok,Chinese Secret:Acupuncture Treatment, 1968.

21. Jang,Yuh Bor,The Handbook of Acupunctural Points 1966.

22. Kim, Chang Kyum,Unique Secrets of Acupunctural Prescriptions.

23. Lee,Byung Hang,The New Analysis of Eight Meridian,1965.

24. Lee, Song Moo,Pictorial Descriptions of Fourteen Meridians in Acupuncture,1968.

25. Lim,Kyon oung,Acupunctural Anesthesia,1972.

26. Ma,Tan In,The Electro Acupunctural Treatment,1967

27. Manaka,Yoshio,"Thum" and Acupuncture,1968.

28. Mann,Felix,M.B.,The Ancient Chinese Art of Healing: Acupuncture,1972.

29. Nagahama,Yoshio,Illustrative Modern Acupuncture Prescription,1971.

30. Russell,Maud,Some Basic Facts:Acupuncture-Historic Background,Theory, Techniques,Actual Cases of Use,1972.

31. Sawada,Yagio,Secret Story of Acupuncture,1964.

32. Serizawa, Katsusuke,The Analysis of Acupunctural Points,2 Volumes,1972.

33. Shanghai College of Traditional Chinese Medicine, Chinese Acupuncture and Moxibustion,1988.

34. Shanghai Medical Society, The Explanation of Acupunctural Points,1969.

35. So, Chung Yu,Case Studies of Unique Acupunctural Treatment,1964.

36. Song,Byung Gee,Natural Medical Treatment: Theory and Practice,1968.

37. Wee, Young Gil,Three-Letter Meridians in Acupuncture,1970.

38. Yoda,Humige,Practical Acupunctural Treatment with Actual Cases,2 Volumes,1971.

INDEX

Ailments of the Abdomen, p.107-133

Ailments of Lower Limbs, p.135-148

INDEX

INDEX

INDEX

INDEX